A TIME OF IGNORANCE AND TERROR

By Brigadier General (Ret) James M. Abraham, P.E.

MY LAYMAN'S EXPERIENCE WITH
SMALL CELL LUNG CANCER

*"WHEN THE NIGHT OF IGNORANCE AND FEAR BECAME THE
DAWN OF HINDSIGHT"*

PO Box 30734
Gahanna, Ohio 43230-0734
614-471-1508
Fax: 614-471-1508
E-Mail: genjima@ee.net

In memory of my wife, Meryl Riley Abraham, her fighting will to conquer her affliction of small-cell lung cancer, to my children, Michele and Daniel, in whose memories she will always be Mom and my hope that the experiences of her futile battle will help someone else facing the same terrible experience.

The information contained in this book has been obtained by the author from sources believed to be reliable. However, because of the possibility of human or mechanical error by these sources, the publisher does not guarantee the accuracy, adequacy, or completeness of any information and is not responsible for any errors or omissions or the results obtained from use of such information. In addition, since the oncologist treating Meryl would not agree to an interview, much of the information regarding Meryl's experiences with the world of medicine are a result of the notes and memory of the author.

Library of Congress Catalog Card Number (Pending)

Printed in the United States of America

Bookmasters, Inc.
PO Box 1039
Mansfield, Ohio 44905-9099

TABLE OF CONTENTS

1

ACKNOWLEDGMENTS

The incentive for this book was the death of my wife, Meryl, and our family's struggle with both the terrible disease and treatment of Metastisized Small Cell Lung Cancer.

The task would not have been completed without the continued encouragement and support of our daughter Michele, son Daniel, daughter-in-law Susan and countless friends.

So many people helped in countless ways. They generously offered comfort, reassurance, and care during Meryl's courageous six-month battle with cancer in 1996. She suffered terribly as the disease attacked more than her infected lung.

Family and friends share my convictions that evolved during our efforts to save her. They urged that I publish the experience, knowledge and information I accumulated as her primary care giver so it could serve as a forewarning for the many people who may experience the same ordeal. Unfortunately, many will.

I also acknowledge the assistance, both personal and psychological, that everyone gave so loyally to Meryl and myself. From the time they learned of her illness until the time of her passing, there was no lapse in their continual support and attention. For this, they have my unending gratitude.

My appreciation to the MD's who consented to be interviewed is without bounds and they will always be fondly remembered. The open arms reception given to me by the various clinics which I visited provided inspiration and incentive. My correspondence with them continues.

The final acknowledgment must go to my dear wife. It was her involuntary suffering and subsequent passing which caused the realization that we are not as advanced in the treatment of certain kinds of cancer as we would like to believe. Those who read this account of a dreadful ordeal perhaps will be more prepared to cope with what they could encounter in similar cases.

If this writing provides them with any degree of knowledge and fortitude, then my effort and Meryl's passing will not have been in vain.

* * *

INTRODUCTION

If only I could have had the attribute of hindsight during the illness of my wife, I believe I would have made a number of different decisions.

Hindsight is always more accurate than foresight because we have the opportunity to learn that which we did not know. Education and experience then replace the ignorance that exists when we face a new and unknown situation.

My wife Meryl and I had been married for nearly 44 years in early 1996. We had been blessed with two children and in more recent years, a daughter-in-law and three beautiful grandchildren.

Throughout our lives, we enjoyed good health along with the joy of gratifying experiences, many excellent friends, and a close relationship that carried us through both rewarding and trying times. Our happiness was such that I only wish everyone could have the same experience. No family could be closer nor could the love have been greater.

An English teacher and school psychologist, Meryl was an intelligent, dedicated and well-educated woman. She had a strong will and devoted her life to help others. When many people were discouraged and forlorn, they would seek her out or she would go to them. She used her strength and encouragement to bring people out of despair.

So many times I saw the brightening of attitudes on the part of those she helped. I also experienced the feelings of gratitude and wonderment that so many throughout our lifetime bestowed on her.

Thus, we were unprepared for the terrible shock of learning in February, 1996, that my wife had contracted lung cancer and that it had already spread.

By the time we were informed of the onslaught of the disease, we were also in effect told that it was too late to do anything. The cancer was terminal.

We became aware during the time she had remaining that despite billions of dollars spent on research and treatment, and repeated statements on progress made against cancer, that conventional treatment still lacked a cure for metastatic small cell lung cancer and offered only possible remission for an unpredictable but short length of time.

Even worse was the fact that available conventional treatment brought on terrible side effects so that any possible quality of life in my wife's remaining days would be destroyed.

Repeatedly, I found myself stating that I wished I had known in the beginning, what I had come to know at the end. More and more, it occurred to me that many others would find themselves in the same situation as ours with little or no idea of what was to come or how to become better informed.

I kept a daily log of events from the time Meryl was diagnosed with cancer to the morning of her passing. This compilation, which consisted of over 200 typewritten pages, serves as an indelible memory of all that transpired. The information which is contained in these pages to follow is not based solely on what I remember, but also on this printed data which was summarized daily.

Meryl's passing has left me with many doubts as to whether we made the right decisions.

When we were informed that she had a tumor on her lung and that there was no cure for this affliction, the blow to our mental stability and the fear that was created were devastating. Perhaps even worse was the fact we were left in a total void as to what to do. We had heard and seen enough about radiation and chemotherapy that we knew these treatments often were worse than the disease. While life perhaps might be prolonged, we felt certain that the resulting pain and nausea would destroy her quality of life.

We also had learned that some members of the medical profession questioned whether, in many cases, a person might live longer with a better quality of life if conventional treatments were refused. Also, my wife had a great fear of both radiation and chemotherapy. Initially she did not want to consider accepting either.

Our entire approach to the problem of her illness was from ignorance, and little or no understanding of what was available or what was to come. It was only after we had lived the terrible days of her ordeal that we came to realize we would have changed what actions were taken.

Except for the fact that the spread of cancer was causing unbearable pain in my wife's legs, I think we would have refused conventional treatment as it was prescribed. I believe we would have opted for radiation treatment on her spine in order to reduce pain-causing pressure on the spinal cord from a lesion. My family and I are also agreed that perhaps we would have allowed only two rounds of chemotherapy, instead of four.

This is not a book of hope or word of a wondrous cure. Rather it is a compilation of what we went through blindly, accepting what we were told and only gradually realizing what was hope and what was reality.

The contents of this book are intended to provide information on the actual suffering and pain that would come as the disease progressed, and as conventional treatments of chemotherapy and radiation were initiated. It is meant to minimize the doubt, hope and the unexpected, where only doubt and hope existed.

When I mentioned to my son, daughter and several others that I was thinking seriously of putting our terrible experience into print, all passionately urged me to make the effort. This writing stems from a sincere feeling on my part as well as our immediate family and friends that the events should be shared for two reasons - realization that as of today there is no conventional cure for metastasized small cell lung cancer and to provide a better understanding of what is certain to happen as the disease progresses.

Information from the National Cancer Institute states:

Regardless of stage, the current prognosis for patients with small cell lung cancer is unsatisfactory, even though considerable improvements in diagnosis and therapy have been made over the past 10-15 years. Therefore, all patients with this type of cancer may appropriately be considered for inclusion in clinical trials at the time of diagnosis.

There is no doubt in my mind that the medical profession will not agree with me and may even attempt to refute some of my conclusions. Yet, I was the one who attended my wife 24 hours a day from the end of January, 1996, until the 6th of September of the same year when she left this world in fear and gasping for breath. Except for the short periods of time she was in the hospital, where I shared the days, I was her nurse, cook, attendant, aide, and comforter for her every need. As she suffered from day to day, I suffered with her and attempted to reduce the pain. The entire family was supportive for both of us.

6

In order to spend the maximum amount of time with her, I canceled speeches, seminars and various appearances. It was my decision many years before that I would never allow her to be placed in a nursing home or other such facility. It was my responsibility to care for her. In other words, it was payback time for all the sacrifices she had made for me and the children during our life together.

Meryl's life touched many and they all remembered. Perhaps the most illustrating example I can share is that after her passing from this earth, person after person expressed how she had been their second "Mom".

This publication is not an endorsement of any herbs, home remedies, or any unusual treatment that might claim to save lives with miracle cures.

The purpose is to promote interest for people to read, consider, question and investigate what might be out there - not to save a life if the life is doomed - but to extend the existence as long as possible with the greatest quality attainable.

If Meryl's story helps just one person, the effort to write it will be sufficient reward.

And if I have found one thought that climbs above all others, it is that, *"The Quality of Life is Much More Important Than the Length of Life."*

What I know now, I am putting into print so that others in the future will not have to state, *"I wish I had known."*

* * *

CHAPTER ONE

THE BEGINNING

We learned on February 19, 1996, that my wife, Meryl, had developed a tumor on her right lung and the cancer had matastisized, or spread, to her spine.

There was no warning, no signs that something was wrong until December, 1995, when she began to experience back pains.

We recognized, however, that the pain and suffering in which the entire family became involved undoubtedly began many years ago when we all urged Meryl to stop smoking. She had started in college and except for a few times when she tried to quit, smoked continuously for perhaps 50 years.

She really wanted to stop smoking but at each attempt, the physical pain she experienced was too great. It was difficult for me to understand why she was unable to stop. Meryl was one of the most strong-willed persons I have ever known. It is only now that I understand that she actually experienced bodily pain each time she tried to stop. She not only was physically distressed, but the pain also caused her to have such a bad disposition that it was difficult to be near her.

Lung cancer was always a remote concern on my part. I was apprehensive that she would become a victim of emphysema and end her days on oxygen, unable to do anything but live from day to day. In the end, the cancer brought about the same condition. For her, the total destruction of any quality of life, caused by both the medical treatment she received as well as the spread of cancer, was heart breaking.

Yet, she clung to life with all her will. Life was precious to her and the thought of leaving this world and her loved ones reinforced her will to live. It was only near the end when she was gasping for breath, unable to eat or drink that this strong will was compromised. Still, the fear of death frightened her and caused me many shed and unshed tears.

When Meryl began experiencing the back pain in late 1995, she consulted a chiropractor and assumed that some treatments would solve or reduce the discomfort. Like many women, she had experienced back pain a number of times during her lifetime and the manipulation of her spine by chiropractors seemed to help. We all thought this was nothing more than a repetition of past problems.

A short time before the pain began, Meryl's dentist told her she needed some extensive dental work, the removal of some upper left molars. Also, she was advised she should consider either implants to replace the teeth or a partial upper plate. She opted to have implants.

At the same time the teeth were extracted, the implants were placed in her mouth. This procedure forced her to spend about four hours in the dental chair. The next day, the back pain began. When it became more and more intense, she consulted the chiropractor.

After more than a normal amount of time manipulating her spine, the chiropractor was having little or no success. As he looked for possible causes, he checked her mouth and realized she had a temporary partial plate where the teeth had been extracted. He immediately placed the blame for the back pain on the dental procedures, stating the problem did not originate in the spine.

As days and weeks went by, the agonizing discomfort seemed to decrease in her back, but her thighs and calves gradually became very painful. The blame for this, too, was placed on the dental work.

During the on-going search for answers, our son, Dan, arranged for her to see an internist in January, 1996. The series of tests the doctor ordered over a number of days culminated with a mammogram of both breasts, a brain scan, chest X-ray, and an MRI (an inspection by magnetic resolution) of her spine.

On February 19, 1996, our final visit to the internist's office, we were relieved at being informed her breasts showed no indication of any disease process.

Shock reverberations came immediately, however, when the internist told us bluntly, "Nothing can be done about the lung cancer."

He said a tumor on her right lung had spread to the spine and Meryl's pain was caused by the cancerous lesion pressing on her spinal cord.

This announcement was made in the most casual manner, not unlike that made over a public address system. The shock left us speechless and in a great state of emotion. The internist went on to say surgery was not indicated on the tumor, meaning it had spread, and it was too late for surgery. We were told a biopsy was needed to determine what kind of cancer she had.

The doctor's words left us with the belief that nothing could be done, that he had announced and pronounced her impending death.

To say the shock was more than I could bear would be an understatement. She was devastated and I was probably even more so. We came home and, for one of the few times in my life, I cried and was unable to hold back tears. Later, I was filled with remorse that I had broken down at a time when she had never needed my strength and optimism more.

While we still struggled to adjust to this fearful crisis, we made an appointment at a local hospital for a biopsy to determine the type of cancer that had developed.

However, one of Meryl's closest friends encouraged her to opt immediately for alternative treatment rather than the traditionally-prescribed chemotherapy and radiation. The long-time friend made several attempts to determine what kind of treatments were available, their locations and the cost. Although without a great deal of investigation, she proposed a clinic in Juarez, Mexico, just across the border from El Paso, Texas.

This search for alternative treatment was undertaken personally by a woman who had become perhaps Meryl's best friend. She and her husband made a number of phone calls, gave Meryl the information, and determined the Juarez clinic was the proper place to go for treatment.

My wife, who seemed to accept without question the advice she was given, told me they wanted to take us immediately to El Paso in their private single-engine airplane. Traveling in this manner would take at least two days under favorable weather conditions, or more if the weather became adverse.

While I appreciated greatly the generosity of the offer, I also was concerned with the time element and the pain she would have to endure, especially if the weather did not cooperate.

It was my wife's wish to accept the offer of her close friends and partly, I believe, for the comfort of being with them. They told us to be ready to leave the next morning, and perhaps yet that day. I was given precious little time to make arrangements to take care of routine matters while I was gone.

We did leave the next day, February 21, but were delayed until afternoon to resolve last minute travel details. Weather had also become a factor. Just before leaving, our son, who had come to see us off, asked me if I thought we were doing the best thing. I told him that while I usually used my head in making decisions, there were times when they had to come from the heart.

My wife was completely convinced that this was the best course of action. She had seen the effects of radiation and chemotherapy in several friends who had developed cancer, most of whom subsequently died with pain, nausea and suffering. Convinced that this type of treatment was nothing more than a death warrant, she believed that anything available would be better and offered more hope.

Our departure from Columbus, Ohio, was into low-lying clouds. The weather had improved enough that we were cleared for take-off. That first part of our flight was fairly smooth, although we experienced light rain part of the time. We were to fly to Oklahoma City, Oklahoma, the first day and go on to El Paso the second day.

However, because of the deteriorating weather, we had to select an alternate destination and opted for Tulsa, Oklahoma. By the time we arrived and found a motel, it was after 10 p.m. and Meryl was experiencing pain in her legs. Worse, her mental condition had weakened and she collapsed into heart-rending sobs. We were able to help her soothe her pain and concerns but by then, it was past midnight.

Our departure was late the next morning. We hoped to be in El Paso by late evening. However, we began to experience very high head winds so that at times, our actual air-to-ground speed was less than 75 knots. With the increasing turbulence, I could see that my wife was suffering terribly. Landing for fuel that afternoon in Lubbock, Texas, we learned the winds were picking up and realized the continued flight would be a terrible ordeal for Meryl. After a brief discussion, we decided to stay over night and hope the weather would improve by morning.

Again that night, my wife experienced pain and mental anguish. All of us did our best to comfort her. I recognize now that the torturing pain in her legs played a major role in fear that she would not be able to survive her illness.

We left the next morning knowing we faced more strong headwinds and our travel would take much longer than normal. The turbulence was even worse than the day before. Air-to-ground speed dropped below 60 knots several times.

Our arrival in El Paso was about an hour late. I had spent most of the flight watching my wife experiencing not only the pain, but also near nausea. We considered it a blessing that she had asked me to obtain medication to prevent air sickness before we left Columbus. It prevented actual vomiting, but not the feeling of nausea.

Because of our delayed arrival, we were concerned nobody would be at the airport to meet us. A driver and a car sent from the clinic had waited for us, however, so no time was lost after landing. We were able to leave quickly for the office the clinic maintained in El Paso, where we were greeted and informed of the health procedures ahead.

Leaving there about a half hour later, we were taken by automobile across the border into Juarez, Mexico. We stopped at a very nice motel where we unloaded our baggage. Next, we were taken to the clinic where the admission papers and forms were completed. Then, interviews and examinations were finalized by the staff doctor.

Meryl's vital signs were taken and treatment, which began that day, included chelation and colonics. The attending physician ordered X-rays and other tests. She also was given vitamins and mineral supplements which were supposed to help build her immunity and physical strength.

Later in the day, we were taken back to our motel where we rested and afterward, went to a nearby restaurant for dinner. This would be the last time my wife would be able to go out. Her appetite was very poor and she ate very little.

The next day was Sunday and the clinic was opened to provide the treatment scheduled for her. I decided to take chelation, colonics and spend an hour in the hyperbolic chamber. I had read a great deal over several months about these treatments. Most of the material had been written by doctors. It seemed like a good idea to take some of the treatments available since I was there and had the time to do so.

I anticipated we would stay in El Paso about three weeks. The time stretched into four weeks. Treatment was delayed because Meryl's hands, arms and even legs no longer accepted the insertion of the needles daily to take chelation. They decided to put in a "port" device that would serve as access for the time she would be there.

Unfortunately, as a result of the procedure, she experienced a partially collapsed lung that night. She was taken to the clinic where they kept her overnight for treatment and observation.

Because of the length of stay, a few problems had developed at home and I had decided to fly back for the weekend. I became reluctant to leave because of the lung collapse, but was reassured the next morning that the problem was not major nor threatening and everything would be all right. So I did leave on Friday, March 8, and returned on Monday, March 12.

The pain in her legs constantly worsened while we were in Juarez. Many nights, I massaged and applied a special salve, with hot towels, to her legs to help relieve the pain. This and a heating pad, which she used constantly, seemed to help. By the time we were ready to return home, however, she was able to take only a few steps on her own and we had to rely on a wheel chair.

Near the end of the four weeks we were at the clinic, the staff physician recommended surgery on the spine to remove the lesion which in turn would greatly reduce or eliminate the leg pain. Our son and daughter were opposed to having this done. Arrangements had been made at a local hospital for an examination and recommendations. However, before leaving, my wife wanted to consult with other doctors who had been recommended to us.

Thus, our departure was delayed by three days while appointments were made. On the eve before our return, one of the doctors actually stopped at our motel room. His advice was not to have surgery because he was convinced radiation was a better choice and would reduce or eliminate the lesion.

We left El Paso the morning of March 19. Meryl was unable to walk. We had arranged for a wheelchair at each stop and at home. While the trip took a good part of the day, she seemed to bear up fairly well. In fact, it appeared she anticipated returning, although she had expressed a fear prior to departure that she was coming back to die.

We landed late in the afternoon on March 19. Our daughter, Michele, picked us up at the airport and took us home. We quickly unpacked and made my wife comfortable in a downstairs bedroom, which Michele had made ready.

That night, the pain in her legs was very intense. I applied the salve and then hot towels. The pain seemed to subside so that she was able to go to sleep. However, the heating pad was placed over her right thigh where it remained the entire night.

And so ended what I have called the beginning, the start of an ordeal which we had to endure far beyond my wildest imagination. What I did not accept then and throughout most of a terrible nightmare was that I was seeing the beginning of the end.

* * *

CHAPTER TWO

Beginning of Conventional Treatment

I believe Meryl was happy to be home when we returned on March 19, 1996, even though she had a great fear of having to submit to conventional treatment.

During our stay in El Paso, we met people who had gone there as a last hope in seeking a cure for their cancer. And it's important now to mention that the attitude and concern of all the personnel at the clinic were beyond anything I had expected. They were more caring, attentive and heart warming than anything I had ever experienced. Such an environment provides the patient with hope and confidence! However, there was very little response from the clinic itself, once we left. I sent three letters, two of which were addressed to the staff physician. The other went to the clinic thanking the staff for the care and hope they had provided.

The doctor, who responded to both letters I sent him, promised to call in a few days. The call never came. We never heard from the clinic except for a flier advising us of a summer special they were having. Thus, while the care they provided while we were there was unprecedented, we had absolutely no subsequent follow up.

The day after we returned from the clinic, March 20th, we went to a local cancer hospital where our son Dan had arranged an appointment. The records and x-rays which we had brought back from Mexico were examined and we were told that a biopsy was necessary to determine what type of cancer my wife had. Even though we had been told the clinic in Juarez would take care of all the necessary medical procedures in the testing for cancer, we were finally told by the clinic doctor that this would have to be done when we returned home.

A bronchoscopy was performed the next day at a local cancer facility by her new doctor. He told us he had been unable to find the tumor and had done a scrape. This procedure is performed by inserting a tube through the nose and down into the lung. With the device, the physician can see the lung and take a specimen from the tumor. Because my wife had been told that the tumor was not actually found, a ray of hope arose that perhaps there was no actual tumor.

The next appointment brought the bad news. The biopsy showed that the cancer was "Small Cell", which is the most aggressive and fastest-growing type of lung cancer. Our family did not want my wife to know this, but the doctor insisted he had to tell her. This news was devastating to her. He said the only hope was in radiation treatments on the spine to relieve the pressure of a lesion on the spinal cord, which in turn was causing the pain in her legs. Also, if chemotherapy was not started immediately, she might only have "two or three" weeks to live.

Radiation began on March 25th and fifteen treatments were scheduled, ending on April 12. While Meryl was violently opposed to both radiation and chemotherapy, the news of her condition frightened her enough that she submitted to both.

I took her to the hospital every day except Saturdays and Sundays while the radiation treatments were in progress. Even while having radiation, she began taking the first round of chemotherapy on an out-patient basis on March 29th. At the treatment center, they gave her the first dose intravenously (By IV). She took the next three doses orally over three days. The final treatment was by IV on the fifth day.

During this time, she experienced a lack of appetite and severe nausea. The combination of both radiation and chemotherapy at the same time had a terrible effect on her, both physically and mentally.

There were times when we had long waits at the hospital because of radiation equipment malfunctions or an overload of patients. My wife became very nauseated and weak during these delays. One day, the wait was exceptionally long and she became so ill that we had to return home without treatment. For the most part however, the waits were short to moderate.

Our oncologist began to prescribe drugs in an attempt to counteract the side effects of the treatment. Narcotic-type drugs were used to help relieve the pain. Other drugs were used to help appetite, reduce stomach acid, and relieve indigestion or nausea. Beginning two days after the last chemotherapy treatment in this first phase, I was taught to give injections and began by giving her the drug Neupogen by syringe. It helps restore the white blood cell count as well as other factors in the immune system. The prescription was for ten injections, one each day for 10 consecutive days.

A critical period is reached about ten to fourteen days after chemotherapy begins. During this potentially-alarming time, which last four to five days, the patient has to avoid all fresh fruits and vegetables because of potential infection. With the lowering of the immune system, the patient is susceptible to any bacteria present in fresh food. Once the immune system is restored, then patients are allowed a normal diet again.

A nurse came to our house three times a week to take blood samples and monitor Meryl's system. As her condition improved, the visits were reduced to once a week. In the meantime, I took blood pressure, temperature and pulse measurements four times a day. I was cautioned to call the doctor or take my wife to the hospital immediately if her temperature reached 100.5 degrees as this would indicate she had an infection and would need to be given antibiotics via an IV.

Also, if the blood platelets dropped below 20,000 or the hemoglobin dropped to 7.5, she would need an immediate transfusion of whole blood and perhaps platelets.

Radiation treatments on her spine were started March 25 and ended April 12. The first round of chemotherapy began March 29 and ended April 2. The 10th and last Neupogen injection was given on April 13. I think we both gave a sigh of relief.

During this time, her physical condition, strengthened by treatments she received in Mexico, returned to normal levels. She began to feel a little better. Her hair had begun to fall out, but she still had enough that it was not too noticeable.

On April 17, we returned to the cancer clinic for an appointment with her oncologist. Blood was taken and she had a chest x-ray. The doctor told us there had been a drastic reduction in the size of tumors, and the first round of treatment had produced dramatic results.

His comment was that she had gotten rid of a lot of cancer cells. We felt our first surge of hope and joy at this announcement. Meryl's spirits were noticeably lifted and she told the doctor she was going to "whip this thing".

I think that was one of the few happy days during the entire time she was subjected to treatments for pain and suffering, which we now know would not and could not cure the disease.

* * *

CHAPTER THREE

Second Round of Chemotherapy
Side Effects and Hospitalization

Our next appointment with the oncologist was on May 8. The second round of chemotherapy began at a clinic with the drugs being administered by IV.

The next morning at home. Meryl began to experience a great deal of nausea. I gave her the remaining treatment orally for the next four days. The doctor advised that I give her another drug daily to combat nausea prior to giving her the chemo capsules.

Although we were able to complete the chemotherapy at home, her appetite disappeared, the nausea continued and she began to develop a temperature. She took the last capsules on May 9 and I began Neupogen injections on the 10th. In the meantime, her condition continued to deteriorate until she would not get out of bed except to go to the bathroom.

Finally, and after talking with the doctor again, I took Meryl to see him on May 13. He examined her and stated he wanted to put her in the hospital. Arrangements were made and I took her there. Even though we arrived at the clinic in the morning, it was much later in the afternoon before we were able to get her admitted to the hospital.

Her stay in the hospital would be much longer than we anticipated, a total of eleven trying days. While hospitalized, she was on IV's continuously, including antibiotics to combat what was believed to be an infection and to restore the water content of her body. Dehydration had occurred during the time at home when she ate very little and only drank enough water to swallow her medication.

At the same time, the amount of narcotics had to be increased to help relieve the great amount of pain she was experiencing in her right hip and legs.

A new problem developed after several days in the hospital when her veins would not accept the IV's she was being given, and swelling occurred where needles were inserted.

We all agreed to a recommended surgical procedure to install a device called a Metaport in her chest. This device had a double port, or entries, so that two needles could be used at the same time. In this manner, IV's, transfusions, etc., could all be administered using the Metaport. We were told this would solve the dilemma which had surfaced because of the situation with her veins.

Meryl continued to receive injections of Neupogen while hospitalized. However, after the first one, her white blood count rose far above normal and the injections were stopped. Within two days however, the white counts dropped dangerously and the Neupogen was started again. Also, her red blood counts as well as platelets dropped to a point where she was given two packs of whole blood and the next day, two packs of platelets.

Finally, on May 24, we were told early in the morning that she had been pronounced well enough to be released. We were ready to leave in a short time but the necessary paper-work had not been completed. It was to be an all-day wait.

Shortly after six o'clock, a doctor came in with prescriptions and the final discharge instructions. One of the prescribed items was a portable potty chair which could be placed on the floor beside her bed. Because she had been using the one at the hospital most of the time, I anticipated it would be needed that same night. I learned in a telephone search that the only store with one in stock would close at seven o'clock. So I quickly left to get there before the closing time.

After returning to the hospital, we reviewed the discharge instructions as well as the doctor's prescriptions. Because the pharmacy was closed by this time, I had to wait until the next morning to have the prescriptions filled.

Meryl needed only three more Neupogen shots at home since the hospital staff had already given her the balance of the ten prescribed. I gave her the remaining shots, with the final one completed on May 27.

Her white counts had returned to normal and she was feeling much better. After she returned home, nurses continued to come to the house for blood samples to monitor her physical condition constantly. Her condition continued to improve and she entered into another period where we all became optimistic again. I took her outside several mornings to enjoy the sun for short periods of perhaps 30 minutes. She would become quite warm and asked to be taken back into the house.

By this time, the hair from every part of her body had practically all fallen out. Not only the hair on her head but also the eyes, lips, arms and legs. Much to my surprise, the hair from the vaginal and rectal areas was gone.

Meryl often wore the wig which she had purchased shortly after being told she would lose her hair. She always wore it on the few occasions when someone would stop by for a visit or when we made trips to the doctor. Her mental condition was still such that she was always concerned about her appearance, even when only members of the family were with her.

The next appointment with the oncologist was on May 4. Laboratory blood work and X-rays continued in the meantime. Her right hip, which had been bothering her, was X-rayed to determine if the cancer had spread or another problem existed. The doctor considered radiation on the hip, but the order was not given. Radiation finally began during her last period of hospitalization when an X-ray showed a lesion had caused a hair-line fracture in the hip.

I was becoming very concerned about the number of X-rays Meryl was having. An important part of treatment seemed to be the constant monitoring of the tumor in the lung. However, X-rays were being taken so often I was becoming apprehensive about the amount of radiation she was absorbing. Although I was told they were necessary and were taken with very low-level machines, that did little to relieve my alarm.

The last act of the second round of chemotherapy was an appointment with our doctor on May 4. Meryl had improved enough that she was able to walk a little with a cane. Most of the time, however, she had to use a walker. We had some dining room chairs at home with casters mounted on the legs. She discovered one of these chairs was easier to use at home than any of the special equipment, such as a walker.

After the doctor examined her, he told us she was showing excellent progress. Her weight had increased from a low of 108 pounds to 126. Her normal weight was 124, but had reached about 140 pounds the previous December. Her spirits were excellent, and she had regained her confidence that she would recover. Blood results were still not up to normal levels, however, and we are apprehensive about starting another round of chemo at this time.

* * *

CHAPTER FOUR

Round Three of Chemotherapy in Hospital

Our oncologist told us during an appointment on June 4 that Meryl's remission of tumors was continuing and she had gotten rid of a lot of cancer.

When we first arrived for the appointment, we learned it had been canceled, but no one had informed us. My wife ended up sitting in a wheel chair over three hours while we waited for the doctor to have a break between scheduled patients.

Our family had agreed that her condition was probably not up to withstanding another round of chemotherapy at this time. I mentioned this to the doctor, who felt she would be all right. Treatment was not to be started until the following week and he wanted her in the hospital for three days of chemotherapy with an IV. He wanted treatment to start on June 11.

When I checked with his nurse, I was told he would have no time on the 11th and it would have to be on the 12th. That was the day I was supposed to go to Washington, D. C., to participate in a special briefing. I canceled the trip and substituted my presentation in written form. I just did not feel comfortable leaving on the day she was to enter the hospital.

We arrived at the hospital on the afternoon of June 12. All the arrangements for admittance had been made, so there was no delay. Meryl's treatments on June 12, 13 and 14 went very well, and she was able to tolerate the IV's with very little trouble. She was released on the 14th and I brought her home early in the evening.

After this round of treatment, I not only had to give her the 10 Neupogen injections but also had to begin weekly injections on Monday, Wednesday and Friday of another drug called Epogen. Neupogen helps build up the white blood counts. The prescription was still the same requiring ten injections on ten successive days beginning the day after chemotherapy is completed. Epogen injections however, were to be

20

given at the rate of one injection every Monday, Wednesday and Friday until her red counts were back to normal. Her oncologist would decide when they should be stopped. According to the information that the manufacturer furnished with the drug, the injections were to be stopped when the Hematocrit level reached 36 percent.

The information was quite lengthy and described many different situations. It also seems that directions, included with drugs and furnished by the manufacturer, are printed in extremely small type. In the instructions for Epogen, it was stressed that regardless of the reason for using this drug, at some point iron would have to be prescribed because a deficiency would develop. Without sufficient iron, the Epogen would not be effective.

As the white blood cell levels dropped, indicating a lowered immunity, fresh fruits and vegetables again were prohibited because of the risk of bacteria which in turn could cause infection. Thus, a natural source of iron was not available. Combined with the expected drop of red blood cell levels, the need for extra iron in the production of new blood is predictable.

After Meryl's release from the hospital, she seemed to improve rapidly. The white blood cell count slowly rose each day and would reach normal levels at the time of the tenth injection of Neupogen.

However, the red blood counts continued to drop. The information from the drug company stated that it would be at least four to six weeks before the Epogen would start taking effect.

As mentioned earlier, an indicator that the Epogen had reached its effectiveness was when the Hematocrit reached a level of 36%. Then, according to the drug manufacturer, the Epogen was to be discontinued. A count of 36% was at the bottom of normal levels. However, it never got quite that high and the Epogen was continued until sometime in August.

Lab results of blood samples taken by a nurse at our home on June 21 confirmed the drop in the red blood count. A remedy for this on-going situation was for her to have a blood transfusion at the hospital the next day. We left home on June 22 at 10:45 a.m., arrived at the hospital about 11:45 a.m. We waited until later in the afternoon for all the necessary tests, etc., to be completed. The staff took a great deal of care to make certain a proper blood match was made. Then the blood was transferred very slowly.

We finally left the hospital shortly after 7:30 p.m. and arrived home about 8:00 p.m. My wife was very tired and went to bed almost immediately. However, she was in good spirits, had a snack before bedtime, was experiencing little or no pain and was asleep very quickly.

When she had reached the critical ten to fourteen-day period after chemotherapy and needed the transfusion to correct the low red blood cell counts, her spirits had declined. Her red cell counts, which were below normal at the start of the round of chemotherapy, had reached a critical level just 9 days after her last day of treatment.

After arriving home following the transfusion, however, her attitude brightened again and she stayed in good spirits for the intervening period until the next round of chemotherapy.

The time after the third round of chemotherapy ended and the fourth round began in July was when Meryl had her best days during the entire ordeal. Her morale rose and she seemed to have reached a point where she began to believe that she was conquering the disease.

She also was more mobile than at any time during her illness. In fact, she was able to use a cane. We went to our son's home one afternoon to visit and she surprised everyone with her suddenly renewed ability to walk.

My outlook also improved, while my conviction that she would overcome her disease reached a point where I was certain we would have many months of better health. My feeling became even more certain there was hope, in spite of knowing the contents of a letter her doctor had written to another doctor. He had stated that except in only five percent of cases, life expectancy was only four to eleven months.

On June 24, I gave Meryl the last of the Neupogen injections. Her white blood counts came into the normal range and stabilized there. Epogen shots were continued as the red blood counts remained below normal.

The Metaport, the device surgically implanted in my wife's chest during the former twelve-day hospital stay, had presented clogging problems from the beginning. It had dual ports for needles, so blood could be taken or IVs injected. It was supposed to eliminate the need to insert needles in her arms. We had no problem with fluids going into the vein, but on many occasions no blood could be withdrawn. Special chemicals had to be used to try to clear the clogging problem. While we had temporary successes, many times blood had to be drawn from the arms. Because of the difficulty of accessing the veins, both arms became badly bruised.

Using the Metaport as access for drugs, fluids and blood still was painful when a needle was inserted into either port because the flesh covering it had to be punctured. We obtained a prescription for a salve which was applied about an hour before the port was used, and this numbed the area to the extent she hardly felt the needles being inserted.

It is distressing to me and I think tragic that some professionals who took blood could do it quickly and with little or no difficulty. Others had poor success and had to pierce her arms several times. At a later time when she was hospitalized again, one attendant had her in so much pain I told the nurse on duty to stop the process. She was piercing her arm time and time again without being able to access a vein successfully. I told the nurse that unless they had someone more proficient, I would not allow any further attempts. Meryl was suffering enough and did not need to be tortured additionally.

A nurse later told me they no longer took blood, that aides now had that responsibility. She also admitted some were not so well trained in the procedure. That was obvious to me.

During Meryl's last hospitalization the decision was made to remove the Metaport. That will be related later. In the meantime, another attempt was made to clear ports in the device using a drug called Heparin. It was supposed to dissolve blood clots which clogged the openings.

Our next visit to the hospital, on July 2, involved arriving early for a chest X-ray and Cat Scan. Except for the time needed to complete the procedures, there was very little waiting and we were home by about noon.

My wife's condition improved very noticeably, so I left for a couple of hours on July 3 to participate in a radio program. Her spirits remained high and she continued to feel better. The next day, I participated in the 4th of July parade wearing my army uniform and riding in a World War II Jeep. Our grandson Riley joined me, wearing his new battle dress fatigues I had bought for him a couple of months earlier at Fort Knox. Everyone was quite excited and Meryl was determined to watch the parade. Our children, Michele and Dan, put her in a wheelchair and took her to the end of our driveway where she obviously enjoyed watching the entire parade.

This was perhaps the happiest day, for her and for all of us, during her entire battle with cancer. While she would still experience days of optimism, good appetite, spending time in the sun on nice days, none of these small joys reached the comfort of that one day when the entire nation celebrated the Fourth of July.

Our family had discussed and decided to ask Meryl's oncologist to let her take a break from chemotherapy. The fourth round was scheduled to begin July 16.

We also had seriously considered the idea of taking her to San Diego for some alternative treatment if she were able to travel.

I telephoned a clinic in San Diego that had been recommended by a local man who had been treated there. He had received chemotherapy before going, and claimed experiencing what he called a miraculous cure. An old friend who had learned of Meryl's illness had called time after time in an effort to get information on what alternate treatment was available. His concern will always have my undying gratitude.

Our son talked with the man who had been treated at the San Diego clinic for his opinion. The former patient said he had gone there with little hope after being told he had a very short time to live. He stated he could only judge by results - he had come back in good health, had no sign of cancer and was working every day. This convinced me we had nothing to lose.

The cost for the proposed twenty-three day stay at the clinic was comparable to a two-day hospital stay in our local area. However, Medicare and many supplement policies do not cover that type of medical expense.

While the cost of two days of hospital care seemed to be given little consideration by the medical personnel, their perception of the same cost for 23 days in alternative treatment appeared to be that it was very expensive.

I mailed a large packet of information regarding Meryl to the clinic so her history and condition could be studied prior to our arrival. We planned to wait until she was strong enough to travel. In the meantime, I purchased vouchers to be exchanged for airline tickets when we felt the time was right to leave.

Meryl was feeling better each day and the red blood cell counts continued to improve. And we allowed the next and final round of chemotherapy to begin.

* * *

CHAPTER FIVE

Round Four of Chemotherapy and Much Suffering

Meryl seemed very responsive to her oncologist during the next appointment on July 19. I sensed they had developed a relationship in which she had reached a point of deep trust in him.

While we were waiting for drugs to take effect that a nurse had given my wife to dissolve clots in the Metaport, the doctor chatted with Meryl and asked how things were going.

Before I was really aware of what was transpiring, he said he wanted to put her in the hospital again for the fourth round of chemotherapy since round three had worked so well. And Meryl agreed, although stating she preferred the treatment as an outpatient.

Her agreement came as a shock to me. It was not what we had discussed.

We had considered the possibility of taking time off before the next, or fourth, round of chemotherapy, perhaps 30 days or so. The doctor was agreeable, but proposed we wait until after the next or fifth round of treatment. Actually, I thought we had all agreed to postpone the fourth round with the idea that within a week or so, she would be able to travel to San Diego for alternative treatment.

On the way home that morning, I asked Meryl why she had agreed so quickly to starting another course of chemo. She stated she did not want to violate the "trust" that had been established with the doctor and we needed to be honest with him about any alternative plans. That was the reason she felt it best to go on with the chemotherapy, she said.

I was not quite sure of that reasoning because if we did go for alternative treatment, we would only be gone for 23 days. She would be able to keep her future appointments as none was scheduled until after that period of time. She felt the doctor should be told well in advance of any plan for us to leave, and he should be told of what we would be doing. In her mind, this was in fairness to him and also so that he could plan his treatment.

Certainly, to do otherwise would not be fair or ethical to the doctor, she said.

I reluctantly agreed, but felt we also should tell the doctor that we had discussed plans for alternate treatment with our son and daughter, and her special friend. Everyone had agreed to going for the 23 days of alternative treatment. However, even though Meryl had agreed, she chose not to do so, but went ahead with plans for more chemotherapy.

I really believe that by this time, she was beginning to get used to the up and down levels of health and life. She would improve noticeably after the ten to fourteen-day critical period after the drugs had been given. Unfortunately, just as she was able to move about, feel a great deal better and start to enjoy living, the time would arrive for the next round of chemo which would destroy all quality of life.

Beginning with the critical period after her first chemotherapy treatment, and with each subsequent treatment, my wife's blood levels would drop below normal. Later, the white blood cell counts improved into the normal range. However, the red cell counts stayed below normal and each subsequent treatment began with the red count still unrecovered. I had great apprehension and the distinct opinion that if we began the fourth round with the low level, I was certain transfusions of whole blood or platelets would be necessary. My fear of tainted blood caused me considerable concern.

What is most tragic is that she did not have the opportunity to enjoy a better quality of life except for just a few days before each round of chemotherapy. She would improve to a point where she could move on her own, even at times without her walker. Her appetite would improve, her weight returned to above 125 pounds and I would tease her about having to cut back on her food. After the first stay in the hospital when they were able to control her nausea and pain, I found that in addition to the normal three meals a day, a snack in between meals and another snack before bedtime seemed to help prevent the kind of nausea she had been experiencing.

One of my greatest regrets is how each period of improvement would be cut short. In my estimation, and it comes from being with her literally 24 hours every day, another week or two between treatments might have let her physical condition strengthen to a point where she could better handle each round of chemotherapy. However, the drug company schedules, the doctor's experience with the effects of the treatment, and the sincere belief that radiation and chemotherapy were prolonging life took precedence.

My wife, who initially was totally opposed to any kind of chemotherapy as well as radiation, changed her mind as the days went by. This surprised me then, but I now understand better why this happened. The relationship and trust with the oncologist gave her the confidence she needed to believe she would overcome her disease. It was my duty to reinforce this trust, as mental outlook and hope play a very important role in recovery from any disease.

The fourth round of chemotherapy was to begin the morning after the doctor's appointment. or Tuesday, and end on Thursday, July 18. Since the Neupogen injections were to start after the last day of chemotherapy, I would begin to give them on Friday.

Although she seemed to withstand the chemotherapy very well, Meryl experienced a small degree of nausea after the third day. I had continued the Epogen injections, to help restore the red blood cells, and was hoping they would begin to take affect so a transfusion would not be necessary.

Previous experience with Neupogen showed that an injection for ten consecutive days brought the white blood cell levels into the normal range and usually beyond. Then, it would be two or three days before they settled down and stayed in the normal range. So there is no question in my mind that this particular drug is very effective and produces the results for which it was designed. However, the Epogen injections had not seemed to have much effect, if any, by Friday, July 19. The injection that day was number 15 or the end of the fifth week of three injections each week. The drug company literature about the drug stated it would take four to six weeks to be effective.

Meryl seemed to improve the next several days. Her appetite again began to gradually return. Each day during her entire illness, I would ask what she would like for each meal as well as snacks in between. When she was undecided, I suggested something I thought she would like and would provide the best nourishment. There was always that critical period, however, when she could not have fresh fruits and vegetables for fear of infection from bacteria.

Within a short time after treatment, Meryl's temperature started to rise. My responsibility to take her temperature, blood pressure and pulse four times daily continued as an important part of constantly monitoring her condition. My instructions still remained that if her temperature rose above 100.5 degrees, I was to call the doctor.

This happened about the fourth day after treatment. Since it was not yet time for the critical period, the doctor did not see any cause for alarm. He told me to give her two capsules of Tylenol every four hours. Although her temperature was back to normal the next morning, she was to experience slight variations. For the most part, the readings usually were exactly 98.6 degrees. Yet, I was not totally comfortable, realizing her temperature had been almost a monotonous 98.6, four times a day beginning with her release from the hospital after her second round of chemotherapy.

Her critical period began on Sunday, July 28, which was 10 days after the last round of chemo ended. Her energy level was much lower and her interest in various small pleasures declined. When the nurse came on Monday, July 29, to take blood samples, problems continued with the Metaport. The first needle that was inserted failed to provide blood. After trying for several minutes, she injected a second needle into the other port. Finally, after having my wife change positions, exercising her arms and moving one of the needles, blood began to flow.

My regular routine was to stop at the laboratory near our home later in the day to pick up results of blood tests. It helped in monitoring my wife's condition. I knew immediately when checking the red blood cell count that it was low enough that the doctor probably would order a transfusion. The nurse called later that afternoon and told us the doctor had issued such an order. I was to take Meryl the following morning to the hospital, where the transfusion would be performed on an out-patient basis.

When I voiced my concern, I was told by the nurse, "It's your call". She indicated to me if any problems developed, that would be my responsibility. I was apprehensive about the constant need for whole blood because I felt at some point it could be tainted and cause new problems. We agreed they would take a blood sample before the transfusion to assess her condition and, if the counts had not risen, they would proceed.

We arrived at the hospital about 10 a.m. on July 30. The test results showed levels had not dropped further except for the platelet count. The doctor felt we should proceed with the transfusion.

The hospital apparently was short handed and they were running well behind, so we had to wait. Meryl sat in a wheelchair over an hour before they could find a room and bed for her. I personally felt the nurse assigned to her was not too careful with sanitation, made mistakes and generally did not give the care to which we had become accustomed on an in-patient basis.

It was to be late in the afternoon before the transfusion through the Metaport was completed. I saw that when the nurse removed the needle, she failed to inject the proper drug to clear the port and prevent clotting. When I brought this her attention and asked why the normal procedure was not followed, she said she forgot. She once more inserted needles into the Metaport to do what she should have done in the first place. There is pain associated with the piercing of the skin, and my wife had been suffering on almost a constant basis from all the needles.

I was suffering with her. It had reached a point where I could almost feel her pain each time her body was violated. We finally returned home fairly late in the evening. My wife hardly ate anything. She had no appetite after the day she had gone through.

Meryl had a slight rise in temperature the next day, but it was normal by evening. It climbed to nearly 100 degrees the next morning. It normalized again when I began giving her Tylenol, but from that day on she experienced either elevated or sub-normal temperatures. Since a variation of one degree above or below 98.6 did not excite medical professionals, I assumed there was no great concern. Yet it continued to bother me that she was having a sudden change, compared to the almost constant temperature pattern of the past. In my apprehensive concern, I felt there had to be a reason.

I discontinued the Neupogen shots after the normal prescription of one injection per day for ten days. Her white levels had returned to normal, after rising to almost double the normal top range. But other immune indicators this time did not climb back to her previous levels.

Throughout my lifetime when anything occurred that I did not consider normal, my first thought was there always had to be a reason. The only thing different this time following treatment was the blood transfusion.

Personally I am convinced a combination of the unprofessional procedures of the nurse plus the possibility of something in the blood transfusion introduced this same something in her body that was not there before. I am very sure those who have been educated and trained in medicine will sneer at my concerns but again, every effect has a cause.

Perhaps the cause was a resurgence of her cancer, perhaps not.

Early Wednesday morning, August 7, I was awakened with a call from her to my second-floor bedroom saying she could not breathe. I rushed downstairs to her bedroom and found her gasping for breath. Not knowing what to do, I boiled water and added a little Vicks salve. She breathed the medicated steam into her lungs and, after about five minutes, began to feel much better. Although Meryl felt she would be all right, I called the local fire department to ask where I could buy some oxygen.

Firefighters, who volunteered to bring bottled oxygen to our house, arrived in about ten minutes and started giving her oxygen at the rate of two liters. Her breathing improved further. They also left us two full bottles of oxygen.

In the meantime, I had called the oncologist and told him what had happened. He arranged an appointment for Thursday morning to have Meryl's lungs checked. She remained on oxygen all that night and until we had to leave for the hospital the next morning. As had happened too often, we found the staff well behind and had to wait almost two hours.

When she was given a Broncoscopy, the doctor allowed me to watch the procedure. First, an anesthetic was given, then a tube with a tiny, lighted camera on the end was inserted through the nose and down into the lung opening. The view from the camera was visible on a large screen and in pictures taken. I was given one of the copies.

The cancerous tumor was causing the breathing problems. The doctor told us it had expanded to the opening in the right lung and was blocking air getting into the lung. Even worse, it was allowing fluid to accumulate in the lung which could lead to more serious complications. The situation was bad enough, but I was somewhat relieved that we both received pneumonia shots in January.

Meryl remained in a hospital recovery room about an hour for observation of possible complications from the procedure. After the tube had been removed, she was given an injection to reverse the previously-given anesthesia. She also was on a monitor to check pulse and blood pressure, because her pulse had risen to as high as 130. During recovery, it gradually dropped and stayed between 95 to 100.

It was the middle of the afternoon when we returned home. Meryl was short of breath and wanted very little to eat before going to bed. She had some soup and juice, and I was unable to get her to take all her prescriptions. She wanted to be on oxygen again that night and asked for

Roxanol to relieve pain. She was experiencing discomfort in her legs although nothing as severe as in the past.

I went to the fire department the next morning, Friday, August 9, to see if they would fill the oxygen bottles. The staff there said they were happy to do so, and assured me they would assist if I called with a need for anything. I would have to do this much sooner than I had anticipated, just hours away, in fact.

When the nurse came for more blood samples, she was convinced Meryl's condition had deteriorated and notified the doctor. They both agreed she should go to the hospital immediately. The fire chief had told me if an ambulance were needed, they would take her on a non-emergency basis, especially if an emergency existed.

The fire department squad arrived just minutes after I called, put Meryl on oxygen, increased the flow until her oxygen saturation reached a more normal level of about 98% by the time they put her on a stretcher. The ambulance left for the hospital and I followed in my car - with a terrible apprehension that everything was out of control.

* * *

CHAPTER SIX

Continuation of Round Four of Chemotherapy
More Hospitalization

My thoughts were filled with frustration at the hospital where I mentally questioned why people who are already in pain must endure even more.

I wondered how much the mind and body can withstand before the will to survive is completely destroyed? How long would Meryl continue to fight when each step only led to more pain, nausea and a battering of the body? There is something crude and barbaric in the application of modern medicine, even though the buildings and equipment were modern, and the personnel seemed very professional. But I had been skeptical for some time about whether so many painful procedures were really necessary.

When I arrived at the hospital to join my wife, I passed the medics who had taken her there. They were leaving but stopped to tell me she had been placed in a room promptly and hospital personnel already had started a series of tests. I thanked them for the help they provided. Their interest and attention were such that my appreciation was without bounds.

When I reached Meryl's room, she was in bed with IV's already started and an oxygen saturation monitor attached to her finger. A parade of doctors, interns, nurses and aides was going in and out, with all of them asking the usual questions. I was prepared as I had brought along copies of a schedule I kept on her medication. Each time prescriptions were changed, I adjusted the schedule to state when drugs were given as well as the strength of each dose.

Traditional questions also were asked about her history - allergies, drug tolerance, etc. All this information was in the computer, yet the same questions were asked by each person who became involved.

I don't know if that was a precaution to verify previous information, or whether people just did not check the information they already had.

An intern, whom I later viewed as an outstanding young man, needed a sample of arterial blood for a more accurate reading of her oxygen level. This entailed putting a syringe into her left wrist and into the artery. It was painful and I was affected emotionally to see the continuation of her suffering as each procedure added more pain.

Was it really necessary, I wondered, to know repeatedly the exact condition of her cancer when the tests and procedures reduced her immunity, caused her stress and was painful most of the time. So many X-rays were taken that I suspected the amount of radiation she absorbed could cause new cancers.

Much is said about the danger of radiation from x-rays but I found no record was kept of how much she absorbed on a continuing basis. It seemed to me that once the program started, it either worked or it did not. If it did not, there was no more they could do anyway.

Meryl had experienced some pain in her right hip since radiation first began in the early stages of her treatment at the hospital. Her oncologist had suggested some radiation in that area, but this had not been done. It would become apparent later that cancer had spread to the bone. Even though X-rays had been taken, they did not show this condition.

The reason this is mentioned now is that shortly after my wife arrived at the hospital, she began experiencing extremely sharp pain in her right hip whenever she was moved or tried to move. This precipitated a series of new tests which were conducted well into the night. Other than that on-going discomfort, her breathing became much less labored. She seemed to be resting and feeling better. I stayed until nearly 10 o'clock. Our daughter, Michele, was still there when I left and our son Dan stopped by later.

I prepared to go to the hospital the next morning with the idea of either going from there to Wright-Patterson Air Force Base to pick up prescriptions or waiting until the next day which was Sunday. Since she was in the hospital and getting constant care, there was little for me to do other than be with her.

It was time to replenish the home supply of drugs. The Neupogen injections had been completed at home but the Epogen shots needed to be continued. I made sure the hospital staff did not forget.

I did not make the trip to the Wright-Patterson base for prescriptions that day, however, because we learned the condition of Meryl's hip and what was causing the problem.

She had a hair-line fracture in her right hip, but in a non-weight bearing area. The fracture was caused by a lesion in the bone. It would heal in time, we were told, but the pain would continue for several weeks until it diminished. She was scheduled for radiation treatments on her hip but not until the following week because the facility was closed on Saturday and Sunday.

In the meantime, radiation was started on the swollen area of her right lung to reduce the tumor that was restricting the opening into her lung and causing her breathing difficulty. I wondered about the Metaport because the area being radiated was directly under the port. The hospital staff said this would not be a problem and the port would not affect the treatment. They failed to respond to my questions as to whether or not the port would be affected.

She had radiation on her lung that Friday, then a treatment Monday through Friday the following week while hospitalized. I stayed with her from morning until night, even though she felt this was not necessary. I wanted to be there for her. Sometimes the intense pain she suffered when the hip was moved carelessly caused her to scream, even though she was heavily sedated. After watching this happen, I made certain when she was moved, she was handled in such a way her hip was not stressed.

Also, there seemed to be no urgency in getting her to radiation and then back to her room. The first day, she was left in a corner after treatment and it was perhaps an hour and a half before she was moved back to her room. I went with her each day after that to make sure this did not happen again.

A week after her hospital admission, her red blood counts finally had risen sufficiently that the Epogen shots were stopped. Her breathing also improved noticeably.

She received a reduced amount of oxygen and was taken completely off oxygen when her saturation level stayed in the normal range without it.

While her breathing improved, she began to experience swelling in both arms. Nobody seemed to notice this so I brought it to the attention of one of the nurses. The IV's were removed after the attending

34

physician was brought in. The swelling in her right arm diminished rather quickly, but her left arm remained swollen for a couple more days.

Tests later showed she had blood clots in her legs and in her left arm.

Doctors decided to install surgically, a filter in the return vein going to her heart, so if a clot broke loose, the filter would prevent it from reaching the heart. Installation of the device, called a Vena Cava Filter, was scheduled and then delayed for my approval on the day I went to Wright-Patterson to pick up more prescriptions.

It was completed before my return, however, as they decided our son and daughter could grant the approval. Dan had Power of Attorney and could act legally in his mother's behalf. She also was completely lucid and capable of making that decision herself, but for some reason the attending physician would not accept her approval. When I returned that afternoon, I was told what had happened and why.

The filter is passed through a specially-designed catheter to the site of deployment in the Vena Cava, which is the large central vein that returns blood to the heart. The clots are trapped in the filter so they do not reach the heart. Blood passes around any trapped clots which normally will dissolve over time.

Another device had been installed by her physical therapist that was supposed to stimulate circulation in her legs. This was to prevent clots forming because she was in bed so long with little or no mobility. They put extra pillows and pads in her bed so her arms and legs were elevated higher than her heart. This was to become a permanent requirement to minimize the possibility of blood clots forming.

The day finally came, Tuesday, August 20, when she was to leave the hospital. The Metaport no longer was serving a useful purpose, so she was to be discharged as soon as a surgeon removed the port.

The surgeon and an assistant came into the room just as she began eating her lunch. Since she had been eating very little and was losing weight, I asked if she could finish before they proceeded. She was likely to have little or no appetite after the removal. The response I received was not exactly a happy one. It was quite apparent they were much put out at my request. We were to pay for that. No one came back until late afternoon, and that was after I made repeated requests.

One doctor came in alone, began laying out equipment and inserted a needle at the Metaport site to inject a numbing drug of some kind. He jabbed repeatedly until it seemed it had become too painful for her to bear. Finally, as the drug began to take affect, she was able to relax.

The doctor asked if I had a weak stomach and I answered I did not. He said the question meant whether or not I could stand the sight of blood. My response was that during my time in the military I had seen a lot of blood and while the sight was not to my liking, my stomach was not affected.

He decided I could stay and watch while he performed his Metaport-removal surgery. First he made an incision which was about the length of the Metaport. After unsuccessful attempts to remove it from her chest, he enlarged the incision. Still, it did not come out easily and he made a number of attempts before he was able to lift it free. Then he pulled out the plastic tubing that was attached to the port and which traveled up the shoulder to where it had been inserted into the vein. There was some blood during this procedure but really not as much as I expected.

The doctor closed the opening with seven stitches, which were to remain for about a week until our oncologist would remove them. Meryl had to remain in the hospital another three hours to make certain nothing unusual developed in her condition. This meant we would leave about six o'clock, and she would be transported by ambulance to prevent the discomfort of traveling in an automobile.

After we received the discharge papers and instructions, the ambulance did not arrive at the scheduled time. When I telephoned, the ambulance had not yet left. After another long wait, I became convinced either the order had been forgotten or it had not been placed. It took two more phone calls before the ambulance finally arrived. We arrived home after 8:30 p.m.

Faced with the problem of trying to get my wife to radiation each day in a car alone with the agony of traveling for her, I asked about the use of an ambulance. The response was that there was no authority to order an ambulance, and that travel really should not be a problem for us.

Meryl was very depressed and had very little appetite the next day, Wednesday, August 21. She ate only a bite of toast and a little tea for breakfast. The only juice she was consuming, despite urgings, was just a little in which the pain killing breakthrough-drug, Roxanol, was mixed. I noticed that morning her hair had begun to grow back. It could be a reason to lift the spirits, but I had a concern that if hair was growing perhaps it meant the cancer was becoming immune to chemotherapy drugs.

Because of the pain caused by the fracture and lesion in her right hip, I had a great deal of difficulty getting her gently out of bed and to the car. Each movement caused her to react sharply from the pain. It took much longer than previous trips. As slow as the procedure was, we arrived on time at the hospital, where she received radiation treatments on both her lung and right hip. The return trip home was no less a problem. After a little soup, the Ensure food supplement and a bite or two of ice cream, Meryl wanted to be put back in bed immediately.

My wife's pain medication had become a constant necessity. Her suffering was one of the most difficult things I have ever had to bear.

The next day was pretty much a repetition of the day before. Getting her to the hospital was even a little more difficult. After her radiation treatments, I was told that there was a problem. The staff had difficulty getting her out of her wheelchair and onto the radiation table. They apparently gave no consideration to my dilemma of getting her out of bed and to the car alone.

After a consultation, the staff decided an ambulance could be authorized to transport her back and forth each day. I was grateful, and disregarded the fact the decision was based entirely on preventing the hospital's staff any inconvenience. Beginning the following day, the ambulance service was provided for the duration of her radiation.

After a visiting nurse had left our house on Friday and had taken blood, the ambulance arrived to transport Meryl to the hospital. I explained to the attendants, a male and a female, the best way to handle my wife in order not to jar her hip. The female got on the bed without taking off her shoes. I thought that she would surely stop and not walk on the white sheets but apparently, she did not give this a thought. I would normally have said something about getting on a clean bed with shoes, but my mental state was such that I could not.

In the process of being moved, my wife's hip was badly jarred and she screamed in pain. I tried to help them because the female was struggling.

They finally got her onto the stretcher and to the ambulance, with the young lady complaining about the weight. In the process of carrying the stretcher, woodwork and walls were badly marred.

After returning from the hospital, I took off my shoes and got on the bed to help from the opposite side. We were able to move Meryl onto the bed without hurting her. We had a great morale builder that afternoon, however, when I picked up the lab report on the blood work and realized her red blood counts finally had risen to near-normal levels. I know Meryl was encouraged, even though she did not feel well. She normally would have received an Epogen shot later in the day but I was told to stop.

Optimism increased. The next two days were the weekend and Meryl would not have to go to the hospital or need any injections. This was a time, I felt, that she would rest and improve. But this was not to be.

On Sunday, Dan brought his two sons to the house so she could see them. She adored her grandsons, and her spirits were visibly lifted by their being with her.

Both boys seemed to want to be as near to her as possible during the entire visit. This was usually the case, but this time they remained exceptionally close.

Perhaps they sensed something we did not. I've often believed that children have a premonition or feeling that is lost as we become adults.

* * *

CHAPTER SEVEN

The Final Two Weeks

Meryl was so confused, she questioned what day it was when she awakened on Monday. She also asked if it was "morning or night."

I assumed her condition was caused by the drugs she was taking for pain. This was a new concern, but we maintained our routine of a nurse arriving to take a blood sample and preparing for the ambulance to take her to the hospital for radiation treatments.

My wife needed oxygen during the ambulance ride when her monitor indicated a low oxygen-saturation level. Then at the hospital, the staff recognized Meryl also would need oxygen at home and authorized the needed equipment. It was delivered that afternoon. She would be on oxygen constantly for her remaining time.

Each day during the week was a repetition. Red blood levels continued to be at low levels until Thursday, when they dropped slightly below normal. I gave her an Epogen injection that evening.

Friday was to be a long, agonizing and traumatic day at the hospital. She had an appointment with her oncologist at 1 p.m. so we waited for him at the hospital after her radiation treatments.

As Meryl lay uncomfortably on a bed in the oncology department, she pleaded several times for me to take her home. She no longer seemed alert, and drifted more and more into an incoherent state.

When the doctor arrived, he announced some of the most devastating developments since Meryl's diagnosis of cancer. The chemotherapy treatments were no longer effective, he said. He recommended another drug called VePesid, on which he had kept a patient alive for over a year.

The doctor also stunned me with the startling information that Meryl had developed large-cell cancer in addition to the small -cell cancer that already had been diagnosed. No one ever explained how or when that determination was made. Finally, the doctor commented he thought it was time for Hospice to become involved.

In spite of Meryl's seeming drugged state, I feel certain she heard and understood everything the doctor had said. When we noticed a drastic decline in her attitude and outlook in the following days, we all attributed this to the belief that she recognized we were being told nothing else could be done.

More pain came on top of all that. I asked the doctor about taking out the stitches in her chest from the Metaport incision. He put a softening substance on the stitches and said a nurse would attend to the rest. About fifteen minutes later, the nurse came in and began taking them out. I think I suffered as much as my wife did each time I saw her react in pain to the pulling on each stitch.

It was to be a long weekend as Monday, September 2, was Labor Day. The radiation department was closed so my wife would go three days without any treatment.

With copies of prescriptions for all the medication Meryl was taking, I went to Wright-Patterson Air Force Base the next day, Saturday morning, August 31, to pick the new supplies. Her red blood cell levels were back to a low-normal range so the Epogen was discontinued again.

While at Wright-Patterson, I return several Epogen vials because the liquid had a mottled appearance. The doctor had told me not to use vials which did not appear normal. They were exchanged for me.

I had hoped that Meryl's reprieve from radiation, injections and ambulance trips would prove beneficial. Her condition deteriorated even more. Although her ability to move by herself was limited, she did manage to go to the bathroom during the night by herself. In the process, she fell and I believe injured her hip further.

Also, she was beginning to lose control of her bowels and could not get to the bedside potty in time. Cleaning up the bed, sheets, floor and surrounding areas added a new responsibility. She had also lost her ability to clean herself after a bowel movement so I took on this chore also. What reduced greatly the amount of cleanup was the fact that we placed disposable pads on the bed, chairs and other furniture she used.

We contacted Hospice and requested a consultation. The city service was brought in first, but the doctor felt another was better. Representatives did not arrive to talk with us until Thursday.

Although radiation appointments continued on Tuesday and Wednesday, Meryl's condition had declined to the point additional treatments were discontinued for the time being. We also were using an inhalator in her room to help reduce her lung congestion.

Wednesday night about midnight, her condition became so alarming, we called the emergency squad and rushed her to the hospital. For most of the night, she was just to lie there. The staff told us nothing could be done because of certain hospital regulations.

Her Living Will prevented any artificial life saving treatment, they said. But not sustaining life with artificial devices, and allowing a patient to lie unattended in terrible pain and suffering, are in total conflict and not logical. What happened to the phrase, "do no harm".

They only took a chest X-ray and a sample of lung fluid.

It was about 6:30 in the morning. We had an ambulance called to take Meryl home. It did not arrive until after 7 o'clock, then we experienced another delay.

The medical technician with the ambulance refused to leave until he had written clearance in case a crisis occurred on the way. I offered to give them whatever they needed in writing rather than have her continue to lie on the stretcher. The night had been long. She had and was suffering greatly. My own feelings were not only greatly stressed but I was experiencing total frustration and anger. I could not help but say to myself that our medical profession totally disregards the patient and what it does to the patient. Some personnel though, especially nurses, seem to understand that what is important is what we do for the patient.

Finally, whatever it was that was needed arrived and we began the trip back home. This only took about 15 minutes but it was well after 8 o'clock before we finally got Meryl home and in bed. The night had been a real drain on me, as well as our son and daughter. How much was taken from the patient after such an ordeal? We in this country have become so litigious and fearful of malpractice that human needs have become secondary to protection and legal defense. Perhaps this is a major reason why many doctors will not deviate from accepted, medical procedures.

Thursday, September 4, was a day when Meryl took only a few drops of water. The only medication was for pain, given to her a drop at a time. She was not swallowing well. She appeared to be in a semi-coma most of the time except for a few times when she seemed to awaken for a few minutes.

Late that evening, She opened her eyes. She asked our daughter, "Am I going to die?"

Michele responded, "No, don't think that way." She spent the rest of the night by her mother's bedside.

On Friday morning, the nurse came to take blood. When she reached the side of the bed, she said in a loud, cheerful voice, "Hi Meryl". My wife opened her eyes, smiled and said, "Hi", then immediately returned to her semi-coma state. I believe she not only looked at the nurse, but also glanced around the room to see who was there. The nurse, deciding it was useless to take blood, remained awhile. She and my wife had become very attached. She had tears in her eyes when she left about 30 minutes later.

Later that day, a representative of Hospice arrived to explain the procedures and responsibilities of that organization. We agreed to utilize their services, although they told us they felt the end was very near.

Meryl remained in a semi-coma the rest of the day. She took no food, and we fed water and her pain-killer medication through an eye dropper. I stayed in the room on a chair throughout the night. The family also stayed overnight.

The next morning, Saturday, September 6, I awakened after dozing several times to find my wife was unresponsive to sound or touch. I stayed in the room while Michele, Dan and Susan came in to see her.

Susan later prepared breakfast and called me to the kitchen to eat. She left to go back to the bedroom and within minutes I heard her excited call to our son Dan. I immediately knew something was terribly wrong. By the time I reached Meryl's side, she was gasping for breath with her eyes open, staring at the ceiling.

The end was at hand, I knew, and for the first time in their lives, my son and daughter saw their father unable to control his emotion and tears. I left the room for just a few seconds, then rushed back in. She had stopped breathing but her pulse continued for several seconds.

We closed her eyes but her left eye refused to stay closed. Dear Meryl, she always did have a stubborn streak in her and death apparently did not change that.

Thus did the weeks and months of pain, suffering and nausea end. I prayed constantly during her terrible ordeal. As the end approached and the pain was too terrible to endure, I began asking the Almighty to either take her or cure her. My emotional stress reached a point where I did not think I could bear much more. Certainly, it was not my own feelings about myself. Rather, it was watching what she was going through. The wrenching sight of her agony built up a huge emotional feeling of sorrow for her in all of us. I did not think that I could emotionally bear much longer, the sight of her in such terrible pain and fear. We learned that a tragedy such as this exacts a terrible price. Meryl left us at 10:35 on the morning of September 6, 1996.

This portion has been the most difficult for me to write. It has brought back the event as though it is happening as I write. I have asked myself many times whether I should have stopped the radiation and attempted to take her for alternative treatment. Also, as I reflect, it seemed that as we discontinued her supplements, the cancer was able to come roaring back.

She made the decision to continue the conventional treatment. I have to respect her choice. Yet, I will wonder from now on if other choices might not have been better, if some of the pain and suffering could have been reduced. There is no way to know.

If we had chosen another route and she had died, then I would have had to ask the opposite question - what would have happened if we had continued with radiation and chemotherapy? What I keep remembering is the letter I previously mentioned in which the doctor stated patients with her condition could be expected to live four to eleven months. Knowing this, would another treatment have been better?

These are some of the thoughts that haunt me today. In time, perhaps, they will fade and allow me some peace of mind. But I will never be able to forget her torturous death. I will never be able to completely forget the gnawing doubts about what we did and those things we might have done.

All this is too late as far as my wife is concerned. But I hope that sharing what happened to our family may provide help, knowledge and comfort to others who may have to go through this same experience.

* * *

CHAPTER EIGHT

Reflections

If stress can weaken a person's immune system and allow cancer to obtain a foothold, I am convinced my wife reached such a stressful point of emotional demoralization and total lack of confidence in herself in recent years.

Meryl was an intelligent, dedicated and well-educated woman. Her life had been devoted to helping others. She was a licensed psychologist, English teacher, guidance counselor and school psychologist. She was blessed with the talent, knowledge and will to help everyone with whom she came in contact.

She rallied her own resources to help the many people that came to her in hopelessness and despair. In the end, I am firmly convinced her exposure to the problems of so many became in and of itself, a disease of the mind. The buildup of the concern and stress after many years of seeing so many problems had to be overwhelming.

This heavy burden and a sense of having done less than she was capable of doing served to condemn her to what seemed to me a feeling of failure and a belief of what could have been. So often, I blame myself for not being able to see that her love of life and joy were gradually being eroded. She did not help me understand out of a desire to hide her emotional state from me.

I believe now that even though we feel that we have a concern and give attention to the needs of others, especially our loved ones, we really do not pay even a minimum amount of attention to reality. Thus, problems begin and grow, and it is only when it is far too late that we begin to understand how inadequate we are.

At a time late in our lives together, I believe Meryl finally was overcome by the accumulation of stress and suppressed emotion. She had kept her feelings inside for too long and they finally reached a point where these feelings became stronger than her will. Adding to her distress were the deaths of her mother and father.

It was during this time that she came to know, befriend and love a woman who was an educated psychologist. Meryl began to confide often in this person as she let out the stressful pressures which had been building up for so long.

They began to attend schools and seminars together where they personally were exposed to counseling and psychological therapy which finally left my wife in a total state of mental collapse. Her greatest strength, her will, was in my opinion demolished. She was unable to hold back tears and cried with the greatest anguish at the least provocation. At times she cried with no apparent reason.

Her friend also counseled her, comforted, and provided assistance to the best of her ability. Over weeks and months Meryl began to respond, and one day seemed finally to return to her former personality. She had regained much of her strong will, composure and strength, which so many others needed.

I have read many times that people have cancer cells in their bodies at various times, but the strength of the immune system prevents them from developing into the dreaded disease. Articles also have stated that the same immunity, however, can be affected by mental trauma.

It was not very long after Meryl's extreme period of stress that the cancer surfaced and began its total destruction.

The friend meant well and tried as best as she could from her own frame of mind and experience to treat the problem. However, it may be that it was the wrong kind of therapy and that what was needed was more attention and exhibited love on my part. I now believe that my course of action should have been to move her as far as possible from all the surroundings which reminded her of those things which had brought on her mental instability. It is now too late to be able to verify one way or another whether things might have been different if I had just understood earlier.

My background is that of a retired brigadier general, an engineer, and an individual who has experienced many different challenges. Except for what I have learned from spending forty-four years with my wife, from the osmosis of knowledge that has permeated from exposure to the practice of her profession, I can lay no claim to being professionally qualified in either medicine or the workings of the mind.

But nevertheless, all this does not prevent me from astutely observing what transpired and learning by assimilating knowledge from others. Nor am I prevented from watching the actions of others, something that has been necessary and important to me most of my life.

If indeed the stress of Meryl's crisis in life did allow the beginning of the cancer, it becomes extremely important to recognize this condition early on and do whatever is necessary to overcome problems inherent to the stress. Perhaps this is the nebulous factor that decides why some are struck with cancer, as well as other diseases, and other people are not.

Meryl also was a smoker for over 50 years which undoubtedly was a factor in her lung cancer. Certainly, there is a firm conviction in our society that smoking is the greatest cause of that type of cancer. Yet, it strikes in all stages of life, both young and old. Meryl was 70 when she was first diagnosed and 71 when she died. Why did she not come down with the disease much sooner than she did?

Could it be that the smoking caused the conditions which, in combination with other factors such as stress, allowed the cancer to develop? And do not intelligent human beings do things to themselves which not only reduce their quality of life, but bring on an early demise?

My guesses and intuition are obviously not scientific as standards now exist. Nor would my thoughts begin to meet the criteria that have been established by the medical profession. But in a society in which there has been virtually no progress toward a cure for small-cell lung cancer, other than if the disease is detected in a very early stage, I feel that my guess is as good as anyone else's.

Too often, I have seen mediocrity becoming a standard for excellence. This has at times, reduced my faith in meaningful progress. And these feelings do not come entirely from my own thoughts, but rather have been stimulated by what I have read in articles written and published by members of the medical profession.

It seems there are many doctors who believe that stress and the weakening of the immune system allows cancer to infect the body. Obviously, this has now become my belief.

The illness of my wife, and her experiences prior to cancer becoming active, should be a classic case of supporting their beliefs and is an important part of why I have come to the same conclusion.

* * *

CHAPTER NINE

Doubts, Ignorance and More Doubts

I have continued to ask myself since Meryl's passing what might have happened if we had made decisions differently. The thought or idea that keeps gnawing in my mind is that instead of four rounds of chemotherapy, we should have stopped after the second round and opted for some sort of alternative treatment.

After each of the treatments, except the fourth, she improved, but almost immediately the next round would set her back again. Perhaps after the first two rounds, had we stopped, even without any other treatment, she might have had an opportunity for a brief period of quality living.

My family had read articles by several doctors who questioned whether in many cases, a person might not live longer and with a better quality of life if the conventional treatments were refused. One article in a doctor's newsletter stated if he ever found himself with cancer, he would deny all conventional forms of cancer treatment and immediately go to a clinic which provided alternative treatment.

I cannot say with any degree of assurance that whatever we did in my wife's case would have changed anything. My fondest wish is that it might have changed the quality of life to something far better than that which she had to endure.

Many in the medical profession will not agree with me and even attempt to refute some of my conclusions. So that I am not misunderstood, I sincerely believe that all those in the medical profession who attended my wife believed they were doing everything possible to help her. My feeling is that even though they knew there was very little chance of even short term remission, still it was the only procedure available to them and the only treatment they were willing to accept as providing a chance of survival.

Yet, I was the one who attended my wife twenty-four hours a day from the end of January, 1996, until the 6th of September of the same year when she left this world in fear and gasping for breath. I was with her constantly Yes, she was the one who suffered the terrible pain and nausea, but I suffered with her emotionally. The stress was great as I watched her and tried to do whatever I could. At the same time, I was feeling woefully inadequate with conflicting emotions. This was difficult to endure and to this day, I have not diminished the feeling that I should have and could have done much more.

The entire family chipped in and helped. Our doubts and ignorance dominated our thoughts and conversations. Our daughter began to survey all available facilities, both conventional and alternative. Our son also looked at various options.

An old friend of mine whose brother-in-law had died of liver and kidney destruction as a result of conventional treatment of lung cancer, called repeatedly to tell us about a treatment available in Mexico. His brother-in-law had gone there on a stretcher and returned able to walk and function. However, failure of liver and kidneys caused his death some six months later.

We learned of an individual who lived in Columbus who had gone through seventeen rounds of chemotherapy, also for lung cancer. He too had gone to Mexico to a clinic just south of San Diego, California.

Upon completion of treatment, he returned home and went back to work full time. His oncologist wanted to give him a couple more rounds of chemotherapy to kill whatever cancer remained. He contacted the Mexican clinic and the staff there agreed he should take the additional conventional treatment. This man has been well and working ever since. When we spoke with him, he stated he knew nothing about medicine and could only judge by results. His non-conventional treatment, he believes, cured his cancer and today life goes on for him except for the memory of what he had to endure during the time of treatment.

As we learned more and discovered that the prescribed conventional treatment was a death warrant in some cases, taking patients to the point of death and bringing them back, we began contacting other medical facilities. We already had our initial experience in Juarez. However, it was our belief that the treatment there did little to eliminate my wife's cancer even though there was no evidence that it had progressed further during our stay. The X-rays showed the tumor in her lung remained approximately the same, even though we later learned it was the small-cell type which is the most aggressive and fastest growing.

And so, we all continued in fear of the unknown, hoping like so many people to find somewhere a miracle that would provide a cure. Also, we wanted so badly to find something that would augment the conventional treatment she was getting. We felt perhaps a combination of conventional and non-conventional treatment might provide a cure or at least, buy some quality time. The uncertainty of what to do remained with us not only until her demise but continues even now.

These same doubts, questions, uncertainties and fears will surely beset all who find themselves in similar situations. Perhaps these revelations will provide some spurring of society to cause the medical profession, drug companies, learning institutions and government to redouble their efforts to find the causes and cure for this terrible affliction of mankind.

Cancer is, by itself, a horrible experience for the patient, family and friends. Doubt, uncertainty and ignorance, as well as having to live in dread of what is to come, should not exist if we are as advanced and civilized as we claim. A disease which seems to have become a business is taking a terrible toll of those who come in contact with it. It is time to provide some peace of mind for everyone.

I also realize, in retrospect, the scope of my total dedication and taking of responsibility for my wife's care from the very beginning. I understand how knowledgeable one must become in accepting this burden and care of love. Thus, it must occur to those who may read about this that many who will face a similar situation may not be able to have the time nor the dedication to be a twenty-four-hour nurse, companion, attendant, cook, dietitian, comforter and, in general, do at home what doctors do in their offices and attendants do in hospitals.

The cost of treatment for the six months or so my wife lived after her condition was diagnosed totaled over $100,000. Life is priceless and should never be determined by cost. But that price provided only a few weeks of life. The quality was destroyed, and suffering, nausea and pain became the way of living for whatever time was left. This seems to me to be the most barbaric condition anyone can impose on any human being.

The circumstances demand total commitment by all family members, plus others. Despite the unconditional giving, it becomes a mental and emotional roller coaster for everyone involved.

I can only say that in an age of rapidly growing technology, of discovery and unprecedented progress, the medical profession has not kept pace. Certainly, there are many new procedures, and technology has provided new instruments never before available.

But what I do not see from the distant point at which I stand is that insatiable curiosity that set off the few medical forerunners like Pasteur, Salk, and Sabin. They and others like them knew and understood the robotic routine of using what is available. But they broke out of the mold of accepting that which should be unacceptable.

I do not believe most doctors would deliberately do anything that would harm a patient. But I also believe something is lost in the process of providing medical assistance through doing what has become acceptable, fearing malpractice litigation, carrying a huge load of patients, and trying to remain emotionally uninvolved.

Acceptable treatment and the oath of, "First, Do No Harm", become one and the same. Thus, the pain and suffering caused the patient are lost in carrying out the procedures which themselves, cause harm and pain. And if the body's immune system is the first and only line of defense against disease, how can a medical treatment which destroys the immune system make any kind of sense?

* * *

CHAPTER TEN

Doctor Interviews

My search to learn more about cancer cures and treatments, even after my wife's death took me in many different directions and to a number of locations.

Fortunately, it led me to three doctors I consider to be pathfinders in clearing the way toward greater understanding that patients need more successful and less harmful treatments than just surgery, chemotherapy and radiation - and to the realization that some already exist.

This chapter will include the comments and philosophy of Dr. Martin Murphy of the Hipple Laboratory in Dayton, Ohio.

Interviews with all the doctors were taped and printed copies were submitted to them for their corrections, additions or deletions. Only at the end of each interview are the author's opinions expressed about these people who have an apparent compassion for human life that is exceptional.

I am very proud that they consented to be interviewed and that they allowed me as much time as both they and I felt was needed for a complete and detailed description of their feelings and beliefs.

For what they have done, are doing, and the fact they were not only willing but seemed pleased I was writing this book, I can only express my thanks and appreciation.

Interview with : Dr. Martin J. Murphy Jr.
Hipple Center
For Cancer Research
Dayton, Ohio

The Hipple Center for Cancer Research, which for nearly two decades has been a leader in research to conquer cancer and keep patients out of harm's way in treatments, has developed an even greater patient emphasis for the future.

"We're here to understand and to develop friendly therapies," is how Dr. Martin J. Murphy Jr., President and Chief Executive Officer, described the refocus of the center in Dayton, Ohio.

The laboratory, which relocated in Dayton from New York City in 1979, has become internationally known as a cancer pathfinder in such areas as cell cloning, non-frozen reservation of human bone marrow, and identification of molecules that control blood cell and platelet production in the bone marrow.

The Hipple center has always had an emphasis on research. Now it will refocus that direction from the petri dish and research bench to the patient's bedside.

"Hipple is in a state of transition to where most of our work is going to end up in people, not in mice, not in cells that grow in petri dishes."

Upcoming questions are whether a procedure, technique or treatment will be toxic, damaging or even lethal to the patient, and if so, why.

"We're not here just to develop new things that kill cancer cells. We're here to develop treatments that help cancer patients," Dr. Murphy explained. " Hopefully we're on the leading edge of that wave. I see it occurring throughout the country."

The center in the early 1980s identified the molecule that controlled bone marrow production of red blood cells. Most recent breakthroughs have been identifications of molecules that control bone marrow production of both white blood cells and platelets. All have resulted in new oncology drugs, but approval by the U.S. Food and Drug Administration and as well as a patent is still pending on the results of platelets research.

What do all three of these discoveries mean to patients?

Chemotherapy can kill tumors, but also inadvertently suppress the bone marrow's ability to produce normal blood cells. Identification of these controls of red and white blood cells and platelets mean patients can be given supplements to rebuilt them - such as Neupogen to restore the white cell count and Epogen to restore the red cell count.

There is a supplement to rebuild platelets which is known as Thrombopoietin (TPO). But it could be marketed under a different name in the future. "The bottom line then often will be that patients who have chemotherapy withheld from them (because their counts are low), will not have to have them withheld," Dr. Murphy said. "Their lifeline will not be withdrawn."

All three of these important research projects date back about 14 years when investigations revealed that patients with a rare disease known as Aplastic Anemia were excreting in their urine, the natural-produced hormone that regulates the production of red blood cells.

These patients are at risk for bleeding to death, are prone to severe systemic infections, and are immune deficient. They often die of complications from their bone marrow not producing sufficient numbers of mature, circulating and functioning red and white cells and platelets.

Studies revealed that the stem cell, the bone marrow cells that are responsible for production of all blood cells, were defective in these patients. For that reason these rare anemic patients excrete excessive amounts of the protein hormone known as Erythroplasia which regulates red blood cell production in their urine.

When the protein was extracted from the urine, the gene responsible for making the protein was identified and cloned. A patent was sought, and it resulted in the drug Epogen.

Similar studies continued on the regulator for white blood cells being excreted in the Aplastic Anemia patients, but scientists were handicapped because there were few patients to study. In this country there is an average of one patient in a population base of 200,000 people.

For that reason, Hipple scientists made an international move by looking far away to China, where there is an average of one Aplastic Anemia patient in 75,000 people. Over a period of nine years, 30,000 liters of urine were collected from these patients and processed in laboratories set up in China.

That research resulted not only in Neupogen, but also the very fragile molecule called Thrombopoietin (TPO), on which two companies are working to produce and patent a drug which will stimulate blood platelets.

That drug could be a solution to patients on high doses of chemotherapy sometimes being at high risk of dying because of uncontrolled bleeding from lack of sufficient blood platelets.

"In the future, Thrombopoietin or whatever name it will be called, will be able to be used conjunctively with chemotherapy to keep patients out of harm's way," Dr. Murphy said.

Another future use of this discovery is that it could result in sufficient banking of platelets to benefit bone marrow transplant patients.

Cloning of cancer cells to determine the effectiveness of different chemotherapy drugs also has been a contribution of the Hipple center to the medical field.

The Hipple staff has collaborated with area doctors in cloning cells from patients' tumors in petri dishes in an incubator.

The different dishes of cloned cells are treated with chemotherapy drugs to determine which is most effective and should be given to that specific patient. By tailor-cloning chemotherapy drugs to patients, critical time is not lost in testing the effectiveness of drugs and the patient is not compromised with toxic or ineffective drugs.

One patient who underwent and benefited from the cloning, but died late last year after a much longer life expectancy than predicted, has been a motivating influence in the Hipple staff and Board of Directors refocusing for the future.

She was the wife of one of the board directors. Dr. Murphy told how two and a half years ago, this "beautiful wife" was diagnosed with a massive brain tumor, the most aggressive form of brain tumor. She was given a maximum life expectancy of six months.

"The last three would be very poor quality, so there were three months of reasonable quality," he said.

Supported by her own "incredible courage" and "the power of prayer", the woman benefited from the expertise of the area's most able brain surgeon and the cloning technique to select the most effective chemotherapy.

Over time, she had three brain surgeries, 30 radiation treatments and very high doses of combined chemotherapies, Dr. Murphy recalled.

"I can't tell you if any one of those ingredients was most important. They probably all were," he said. " They brought about a long-term cushion of duration of over two and a half years."

The woman died in December, 1996, of complications, not of the brain tumor, but of serious complications probably from radiation and toxic side effects. She had several serious seizures, but did not recover from the last one.

Dr. Murphy said as a result of her death, a new strategic focus was discussed during a meeting of the Hipple staff members, the surgeon, neurologists, and board member.

"We all witnessed the frustration," he said, "what we have done to patients and what we have done for patients, and sometimes they are so interconnected we can't do for the patients without doing to the patients."

The new approach will be removing the "to the patients" and emphasizing the "for the patients", he said.

"It's a whole new strategy and it means breaking some molds, opening some doors and windows," he explained.

The goal, he said, is not for a surgeon to remove portions of a patient's brain and leave them living but not alive. But to be able to say to the patient, this tumor will not kill you, Dr. Murphy explained.

"That's what our job is," he said. "And in not killing, you are going to have a qualify of life that is going to enable you to retain your dignity as a human being."

Chemotherapy, surgery and radiation have become the three principal weapons to treat cancer because historically they came along first, Dr. Murphy said. Greeks were the first to use surgery to remove cancerous breasts, and chemotherapy developed as a consequence of chemical warfare substances in World War II.

"There was a huge wave of chemotherapy, and the birth of oncology and radiation therapy, and all this blowing it up, and cutting it up and poisoning it," he said.

Dr. Murphy compared this to Mark Twain's comment, "When all you have is a hammer, the world is full of nails that want hammering."

"We have radiation, surgery and chemotherapy. When all we have are these hammers, we see only nails that want pounding. So let's go pounding, let's use them, what else do we have?" Dr. Murphy said. "But we need not just hammers. We need a whole set of new tools so you don't just go hammering."

These new tools are what Hipple will seek in the form of friendly medicine.

"Finally we're saying wait a second, and now the sophistication of molecular and biological hammers are coming to the fore," he explained.

Answers hopefully will lie in molecular science and genetic technologies, he predicted. For example, the same factor that stimulates production of white blood cells also stimulates the immune system. If the gene for this factor could be inserted into the DNA of a specific virus that would carry a killer gene into a cancer cell, it could kill the tumor cell and trigger an immune response at the same time.

"We are working on that now," Dr. Murphy said.

Every person develops cancer cells at some time, and they can proliferate until they clone and become the base of a tumor if left unchecked by the body's immune system.

Yet two out of three people will not get clinical tumors because of their immune system function. The issue scientists wrestle with is how is it that the immune system is so well tuned that it is able in most of the people most of the time to keep them free of tumor cells that are continually emerging, regardless of lifestyles.

The reasons can be multi-factorial, but Dr. Murphy believes an answer will be found and become an improper function of the immune system so that the tumor cell will be unable to mask itself as a normal cell.

"What we need to find out is what kind of determinants are different for that particular tumor cell that is not recognized versus a tumor cell that is recognized by the immune system," Dr. Murphy stressed. "The immune system is not clearly foolproof, it can be fooled. Cancer cells have almost an infinite repertoire of different faces it can put on, and it would be hard to design even in the most perfect of systems, a system that always would be able to recognize an infinitely changeable malignant cell."

Care has to be taken, however, in dealing with the sophisticated immune apparatus not to prompt the system to not recognize a normal cell, or the body could engulf and destroy itself.

Dr. Murphy said advancements are needed in the practice of medicine, but he compared the magnitude of this to changing the navigational course of a super tanker. It can be done, but it takes time. The superstructure of the tanker can not stand a quick adjustment.

"Laboratories like ours are extraordinarily agile. Our job is new ideas, new knowledge. That's why we get up in the morning, hopefully to produce a new piece of data. Whereas in the practice of medicine, there is a conservancy there where one does not want to err and the aspect is not to do harm."

While laboratories are moving quickly, Dr. Murphy sees the need to shorten the time of discovery, application, and clinical deployment. He also sees the need for more funding nationally to advance both discovery and application of more friendly medicines and treatments. Although the Hipple Center should be expanding to expedite new technology, it is downsizing because of finances.

On the issue of alternative anti-cancer methods to chemotherapy, radiation and surgery, Dr. Murphy said his stand is whatever helps the patient.

"It may work by killing the cancer, it may enhance the patient's own immunity, it may in fact add some ray of hope psychologically and provide buttressing support, " he said. "If it is helpful, not because you are selling a commodity, but because there is some basis in fact for the support of the patient, you can't help but encourage that. I may not understand it, but that does not mean I can not believe it or probe it."

Unless a theory is proposed by a known charlatan, Dr. Murphy said he keeps an open mind. He told how Hipple scientists learned in China of traditional medicine practiced for centuries involving a fungus derived from the larvae of the silkworm. It would be considered "alternative' medicine by western standards, he said.

Dr. Murphy's vision for the future is in molecular biology advancements for more human, friendly and increasingly-effective therapies against cancer.

"Not," he said, "in the next generation of anti-cancer chemotherapies, not by the next generation of new sophisticated radiation or better manipulation of surgery. They will all be relegated to the history books and looked upon as barbaric."

People will look back in horror, he predicted, although maybe not in his lifetime, at patients who had massive chemotherapy, radiation, and had undergone mutilating surgeries.

"Our effectiveness has surely increased today, and we've been more humane in the actual administrations of therapy, but the consequences we see as a result of the effects still are totally unacceptable," he said. "But that ought not be what we want to pass on to our children and our children's children as the medicine of the future. It will be far more sophisticated."

* * *

Initial Telephone Interview with:
Dr. Martin J. Murphy Jr.,
President and CEO
Hipple Center
For Cancer Research

My first contact with Dr. Murphy was by telephone and was intended to merely arrange for an interview at a later time. However, the content of that conversation was enlightening and educational. The following is a general summary of our discussion.

I was informed by Mrs. Irene Wright, a former medical reporter with the Cincinnati Enquirer for a number of years, that you have been cloning cancer cells and testing drugs against them. She suggested that I call you and arrange an interview if you would be willing.

My knowledge of Mrs. Wright came about through a number of occasions when she interviewed me on military matters and I found she had a degree of integrity which was unique. She suggested I should get some ideas from you about what is being done, opinions you might have and whatever contributions you would care to make.

My book is essentially finished, I told him, and I think this chapter of interviews would be icing on the cake.

Dr. Murphy expressed his appreciation and respect for the accuracy and integrity reflected in the articles resulting from interviews he had given to Mrs. Wright. He said that he would be happy to discuss contemporary conditions and prospects for the future in terms of research. .He needed additional time because of a very busy schedule, and thought an interview could be scheduled the following month. He said he also would be pleased to read and make comments on the manuscript itself.

The body of research on-going right now, Dr. Murphy explained in our conversation, in small cell as well as non-small cell lung cancer is really voluminous. The NCI (National Cancer Institute), if you have not yet contacted them for their research protocol and of course they are all available to you, would be something that you ought to do. That would be a reference obviously that I'm sure that you will include in your book anyhow for patients to contact the NCI. In particular, an important source is the PDQ,(Physicians' Data Query), which is becoming very quickly, one of the world's most important repositories of all investigational therapies and all clinical trials ongoing. This is not only in the United States but also increasingly abroad as a result of the Internet.

It is accessible to anyone, you or anybody and it is becoming a very important aspect .If your book is read five years from now, all the kinds of commentary that I or anybody else would make would be very outdated. Yet, the numbers will most likely still be intact. That is the importance of contacting the NCI and PDQ for up to the minute or certainly up to the month clinical trials.

The other thing that is happening, as I'm sure you are well aware, is the increasing traffic of patients as well as their loved ones on the Internet in chat rooms dealing with organ-specific disease.

Dr. Murphy told me that previously he was asked if he would be a medical commentator on a number of organ specific cancers, and agreed to do so for such areas as Hodgkin's Disease, Leukemia, Breast Cancer, etc. Within the next 18 hours, he received over 700 pieces of mail. Perhaps 100% of those were patients and patients' loved ones. That's the intensity of the lay person on the World Wide Web in organ specific tumors. He said he finally had to, what they call, unsubscribe himself from so many because he simply could not handle it.

I interrupted Dr. Murphy saying he must have been inundated. His response was, "Absolutely". He said he monitored a number of them, including Hodgkin's Disease. In just one month, he said, there was from thirty to seventy new pieces of communications on the World Wide Web everyday in just that disease alone. And that is in just one chat room, he pointed out. There are multiple chat rooms like this. He added, "I should also say that physicians, and not surprisingly, are the last to get on the Web. For lots of reasons, not the least of which is that they have graduated and they are not all that user cordial and happy on the Web. They don't know what they are doing and they are not alone.

And that's because it's still, the Internet that is, not tricky, but it wasn't as easy as it is now becoming.

"The other thing is just time. A busy oncologist, and I don't know if there are any non-busy ones, but an oncologist will generally be seeing anywhere from thirty to forty patients a day, making rounds and just trying to stay afloat. It's problematic for them to find the time to sit down and sort of explore the Web. Whereas, a patient or a patient's loved ones will make time, as you well know. It becomes these things around which their lives then are centered.

If someone says there is information and plenty of it, there is also some poor information. But there is a lot of good information on the World Wide Web. Patients are going there by the droves. What then happens is that they appear in the doctor's office the next morning and say, doctor, what do you think about..... And the doctor says, `Where did you find out about that?' Then they say, `The World Wide Web.' And a lot of doctors are buying computers because the patients are driving them crazy. That's good, I mean that's good because the more information, the better."

Dr. Murphy then stated, "And now, you are going to be contributing too and I would suggest that whatever publisher you pick, make certain that it gets on the Web. You are going to get an awful lot of people making inquiries about it if it goes out over the Web. I told him I already had received two inquiries from people who are set up to do exactly that and wanting to know if I would consider showing them what I have and letting them handle the information on the Web.

"Before you publish the book, search a couple of those chat rooms. I have been pleasantly surprised at not only the extent of the information, but the depth at times to which it is available."

Dr. Murphy continued by saying, "That is something I would encourage because you will find a lot of patients in the future are going to go there to get information. And the Web will take them to the NCI, PDQ, to clinical trials, the pros and the cons. It will take them into new drugs which are being used as well as those which are just in development.

There are whole new colonies of therapy which include of course, medical anti-bodies, gene therapy and targeted types of radiation that will be much more specific and far less damaging to non-tumorous tissue.

"All of that is happening right now," he said. "It's not as if we have to wait six months or six years. It is in the process as we speak, of happening."

I commented to Dr. Murphy that I was interested in what Mrs. Wright had told me about the research he was doing. She had written several articles about activities and research. Also, I had a very great interest in his work of cloning cancer cells and the application of various drugs to those clones.

In response, he said, "I believe, yes, what we have been doing for some time is being able to clone human tumors, obtained from surgery, from patients obviously who are undergoing some sort of either diagnostic or therapeutic regimen. These cloned tumors are cloned by technology which we helped develop. Then, against them, we can test a whole spectrum of anti-cancer drugs, both of a conventional variety, such as your wife experienced, as well as investigational drugs to which any given patient might normally be subjected. This is only because conventional therapy would have to be employed first.

"What happens, however, is by doing it, by testing a clone of a patient's tumor against a spectrum of drugs, we are able to identify at the outset, which tumors are likely to respond to a particular drug or a regimen of drugs and more importantly, which tumors are not going to respond to a given drug. We can therefore, eliminate the 'no-hope' drugs right up front, those drugs to which the tumor is going to be resistant and the degree of assurance is better than 90%. In other words, if it does not work in one of the clones, it is not going to work in the patient."

Dr. Murphy's next comment had even more impact. "If a tumor we have cloned has been killed by a given drug, chances are about seventy percent that the patient is going to respond to that drug favorably by decreasing the diameter of that tumor by at least fifty percent after one course of chemotherapy.

"It is very helpful to eliminate the no-hope drugs and to maximize the probability of getting the right drug. In addition to that, it sometimes helps patients enrolled in clinical trials where a tumor is found to be resistant to all conventional drugs by then testing it against a spectrum of non-conventional, if you will, investigational compounds.

Chances are that we at least have a better chance by being able to enroll in a more appropriate trial."

Dr. Murphy then referred back to Irene Wright's several interviews and articles, and stated cloning was one of the areas with which she had familiarity. He complimented her by saying that he knew that in past years, she had written some wonderful articles, both on the scientific basis for that kind of assay as well as a number of celebrated clinical cases. In particular, one case of a young lad who had a very aggressive tumor which was brought into clinical remission was at least a partial result of being able to clone the tumor, and identify an unusual combination of drugs which ultimately helped him.

As we made arrangements for me to contact Dr. Murphy's secretary to arrange an appointment that resulted in the interview on the previous pages, I marveled at how much material he had provided in just our telephone conversation.

* * *

Author's Note:

Dr. Murphy's attitude, concern, dedication, appreciation and understanding of the need to preserve the quality of life are emotionally touching.

His comments to the effect that today's methods will be relegated in the history books as barbaric will be understood by everyone who has gone through the trauma of contemporary, acceptable treatment of cancer today.

I am firmly convinced that in his beliefs and comments, he has a real understanding of the "First, do no harm" tenant of the medical profession.

My empathy for Dr. Murphy has developed and grown during our interviews. My understanding of his tremendous concern for people brings about a great warmth and appreciation of this gentleman.

His sincerity and dedication have been, are and will be a boon to the advance of medicine. Perhaps in the future, the profession of medicine will embrace the new philosophy of the Hipple Foundation which is to focus on what is done for the patient rather than what is done to the patient. But we exist in an age where there is too much concern for effect and not enough for the cause.

Only those who develop the mental compassion and understanding of Dr.Murphy will provide the impetus that may accelerate the snail like progress that exists today.

* * *

CHAPTER ELEVEN

Interview with: Dr. Philip E. Binzel Jr.
Washington Court House, Ohio

Poor results in cancer survival rates are continuing in this country because the medical profession is "treating the wrong thing", believes Dr. Philip E. Binzel, Jr., a long-time general practitioner in Washington Court House, Ohio.

Dr. Binzel, author of the book, "Alive and Well", said that "With all our efforts to destroy the tumor or reduce the size of the tumor, we are treating the wrong thing while the thing we should be treating is the body's defense mechanism."

He believes people become unable to fight off cancer cells because there is a breakdown in their immune system, basically because of a nutritional problem. His stress is on a nutritional approach to rebuild patients' bodies and help them resist the disease.

Dr. Binzel is convinced that in conventional treatment, only the symptoms are being treated. Anything in the way of chemotherapy will destroy cancer cells. But they are not getting to the cause. It's like someone with appendicitis. Patients complain of pain so they are given Demerol or some other pain reliever. Then, in about three or four hours, the drug wears off and the pain is back again. It can be said that the right pain medication was not used. But it is not the pain medication that is the problem. The problem is that the treatment did not get to the cause of the disease.

"We give too much attention to the tumor and no attention at all to the defense mechanism and the cause which is why did that individual get that disease in the first place," he explained.

The life threat to the patient is not the initial cancer, but rather its spreading to the rest of the body, Dr. Binzel said.

"The only thing known to mankind to keep that disease from spreading is for the defense mechanism to once again function normally," he said.

The medical profession has made tremendous progress in the last 50 years in the ability to surgically remove malignant tumors, to use radiation to shrink or destroy tumors, and in the ability to use chemotherapy to remove or reduce the size of tumors.

Despite these three forms of preferred treatment by most doctors, Binzel contends the survival time of a cancer patient today is no greater than it was 50 years ago.

"We've gotten so tumor oriented, we ask, `What about the tumor?'. Nobody ever says, `How is the patient doing?' How the patient is doing is the final check."

Cancer treatment today generally is directed at removing the symptom, much like giving a pain killer for the discomfort of appendicitis, Binzel repeated. In the same manner, chemotherapy will destroy cancer cells, but it does not address the cause of the disease.

His approach to cancer treatment dates back to about 1974 when he viewed a film, "A World Without Cancer" by a well-known and respected friend, G. Edward Griffin. But the documentary included statements about nutritional cancer treatment and the use of Laetrile that Dr. Binzel questioned.

"I thought this doesn't sound right, and this doesn't sound right," he said. "But I had known Ed Griffin a number of years, and I was aware he had never ever written or published anything that he had not researched to the final degree."

That was the start of Dr. Binzel's search to learn more about alternative medicines to surgery, chemotherapy and radiation.

Literature was scarce in this country, but Dr. Binzel learned of an organization in California that specialized in gathering and translating articles throughout the world on a given subject.

"I was interested in Laetrile, nutrition and how they related to cancer. About six months later, I got this stack of material. It took me six to eight months to go through it," he recalled.

At that time, Dr. Binzel had been a family doctor about nineteen years and was unhappy with results he was getting with cancer patients.

"I treated all my patients like everyone else -surgery, radiation and chemotherapy," he said. "I had about the same results as everybody else, most of my patients died. I realized that was not the answer, but I didn't know what the answer was."

The articles gathered and sent to him from the California agency included study results among others by Dr. Dr. Ernest Krebs Jr., Dr.

Hans Nieper of Germany, other European doctors and Dr. Ernesto Contreras of Mexico.

"I was convinced that what they said made sense. What we are dealing with is basically a nutritional problem," Dr. Binzel said. "They were able to prove that the body did have a normal defense against cancer, they were able to show how the defense mechanism functioned and that removing the tumor or destroying the tumor does not do the job."

Up until that time, Dr. Binzel recalled, a guaranteed cure for cancer seemed to come down the road every decade - but most were as frivolous or made as little sense as "burying a sock under the tree".

"So I read the works of these other doctors and realized this is where it is," he said. "There was also the fact that we had six children and a dog, and every time the dog got sick the vet would say, 'What has this dog been eating?' It only took me 12 years to catch on to that."

"So I considered that and looked at the medical data, and I said, Yes, this is the reason we have such poor results in what we're now doing, because we're treating the wrong thing. We're treating the tumor. What you have to correct is the defense mechanism - put into that body the things the body needs in order to allow that defense mechanism to function and take away from that body the things that are detrimental to the defense system."

He began using nutritional therapy and Laetrile with positive results, but came under attack for his work.

"It was a constant battle with the state medical board, the FDA (Food and Drug Administration) and so on," he explained, "But I got used to that. Fine, I thought, let's take this to court. At any time I could take 75 to 100 patients to court. And they knew that. They backed off."

Dr. Binzel includes statistics in his book that showed the survival rate of his patients - those who were treated for primary cancer (in one area) before they had chemotherapy or radiation, and stayed on the program, had a survival rate of 87 percent for over five years. He compared that to what he said was the current American Cancer Society's five-year survival rate of 15 percent.

Laetrile, which is considered to have properties to break down a defensive protein lining around a cancer cell, was only part of the nutritional treatment. But the FDA apparently reacted to unfavorable study results in which Laetrile was given to patients who already had undergone extensive chemotherapy and radiation.

"They were still going downhill. They gave them a few shots of Laetrile and said, `Why, gee, they died. It didn't work'," said Dr. Binzel.

Controversy also surrounded the allegation that Laetrile contained a toxic cyanide, but it actually contains a cyanide radical that is a totally different compound, Dr. Binzel countered. It would be similar to comparing pure sodium, a highly toxic substance, to the table salt compound of sodium chloride, he explained.

"Laetrile is simply part of a total nutritional program. Dr. Nieper in Germany has probably done more work along this line than most of the others and he tells us there can be up to 26 to 28 deficiencies in a cancer patient," Dr. Binzel said.

These could range from deficiencies in pancreatic enzymes, magnesium, selenium, zinc or other substances.

"Any given patient can have four, six or ten of these deficiencies," Dr. Binzel said. "The most important thing Dr. Nieper has tried to get through to us is that if you do not correct all of these deficiencies, you are not going to help that patient."

The medical profession is used to looking at chronic metabolic diseases as single variable diseases. Examples are scurvy, pernicious anemia, or diabetes. Cancer is a multiple - variable disease, and unless you correct all those variables, you are not going to help that patient.

He compared all the variables needed to what it takes to run an automobile engine - such as the battery, carburetor, sparkplugs and gasoline.

"It's not a matter of which is most important. Each of these in its own way contributes to the normal function of that automobile. That's the way with Laetrile. But even though the FDA got off on this thing of Laetrile, I used far more of the pancreatic enzymes and Vitamin C."

Generally by the time Dr. Binzel began seeing cancer patients, they already had undergone surgery, chemotherapy and radiation. He started them on a nutritional program, although realizing there is nothing in nutritional therapy that is going to make any tumor eventually disappear.

"Once a tumor is well formed within the body, the body will begin to treat that tissue as normal tissue without attacking it,' he explained.

No tumor is ever more than 10 percent cancer cell, meaning a highly malignant cell, an undifferentiated cancer cell. The other 90 percent cells of the cells in the tumor are basically normal cells - or transitional cells that while they do show effects of cancer, they retain enough of their size and shape that you can identify the tissue from which they come. These are basically normal cells. The body will not attack them.

"Assuming the body will go in and kill off the highly-malignant 10 percent of cells, where this is done it will leave scar tissue," Dr. Binzel said. "The body will not attack the transitional cell, thus the tumor will remain. We keep looking for something to make the tumor go away, well the tumor is not the problem."

He recommends only three circumstances when tumors should be removed:

• Because its size and shape are interfering with a function. If a patient has a tumor in the large intestine that is causing an obstruction, something has to be done or the patient could die.

• If it's size or position is causing a great deal of pain. A patient can not survive indefinitely on strong pain medication.

• If a patient is suffering psychologically from the knowledge of having a potentially-fatal cancer, removal of the tumor may help a person's mental outlook.

• "Otherwise, don't really worry about the tumor, " Dr. Binzel said. "Generally, if the tumor is easily accessible, take it out. It's one less thing for the body to cope with. When you have to go down in the lung and take out three-fourth's of the lung, and the tumor is not doing anything, leave it alone."

Dr. Binzel also believes the medical profession is not dealing with different types of cancer, but with cancer in different parts of the body. If highly-malignant, undifferentiated cancer cells are taken from the breast, prostate or kidney and put side by side, he contends there is not a pathologist in the world who could tell the difference.

"While the transitional cells show the effect of cancer, you can identify that tissue," he said. "But they are not the ones that cause the problem. The ones that cause the problem are the undifferentiated cells."

He also is convinced that whether tumors are rapidly growing or slow growing has nothing to do with the type of cancer, as much as it has to do with the defense of the immune mechanism of the patient. If the immune mechanism is functioning fairly well, then the tumor will grow slowly. If the mechanism is completely broken down, then it will grow very rapidly.

"The more I see of this, the more I am convinced it doesn't have to do with the type of cancer or where it is. It has to do with the defense mechanism."

Unfortunately there is not yet a method to analyze deficiencies in patients' bodies that make them susceptible to cancer, although Nieper has done some work on this in Germany.

"There is the area where the answer lies," Dr. Binzel explained. "If we can take a given cancer patient and draw some blood, and say you are deficient in this and this, and give those items which are deficient to the patient, fine. What we are doing now is using the shotgun approach."

Nutritional programs include dosing patients to make up for whatever deficiencies exist. However, problems caused by overloading patients have to be avoided.

"The body then uses its energy to get rid of the excess rather than fighting the disease you are fighting. So its not a matter of a little is good, then a whole lot more is a whole lot better," he explained. "For example, you can get into Selenium toxicity and Vitamin E in excessive doses."

In order to avoid reverse effects, Krebs and Nieper developed a program to assure that patients would get adequate amounts without overloading them, Binzel said.

The ideal treatment procedure for Dr. Binzel is to have a patient who has not yet undergone chemotherapy or radiation. The initial conference begins with a nearly two-hour discussion on diet, vitamins and enzymes.

"My whole point with the length of time I spend with people, is to make sure they understand," he said. "It would be a very simple thing if patients walked in and I gave them a list of vitamins and enzymes I want them to take, and say here's a diet I want you to follow. Good bye."

That probably would work for about a week, he said. The patients would begin substituting one item for another in the diet, and would be back to the former eating habits in about two weeks.

"The most important part is that patients understand why it is that they must do some things and must not do other things," he said. " Once they understand what is going on, then you don't have any trouble. Most of the time I spend is teaching. It's not so much what I want them to do, but why I want them to do it - what's going on with the body."

Prevention, Dr. Binzel believes is a matter of being on or getting back to a proper diet. People are eating too much processed foods, and should eat more raw fruits and vegetables.

"There are some enzymes in fruits and vegetables that are tremendously important to good nutrition," he said. "Any temperature over 130 degrees will destroy all the enzymes in fruits and vegetables, so you have a problem with everything that is canned, bottled or cooked."

People also need to consume foods with less animal protein and more vegetable protein, because the body's requirements to digest the former helps deplete it's defenses to fight cancer.

"The body couldn't care less for the source of its protein. You don't have to have meat, you do have to have protein. The protein is made up of eight essential amino acids. It doesn't mean people can't have any meat at all. Yes they can! But they should get more and more into the vegetable protein."

A meal of bean soup and corn bread has all the essential amino acids (essential components of the diet) and the body does not have to break them down. A meal of beans and brown rice is complete in the way of protein, while whole grain bread and nuts have all the necessary amino acids.

There are hundreds of foods that can help build the body's line of defense, including strawberries, blue berries, blackberries, Lima beans, bean sprouts, and others.

But Dr. Binzel said in the four years he was in medical school, the year he was in internship, and during his year of residency, he never heard a single lecture on nutrition.

He personally believes this is because drug companies, which profit from the sale of drugs for cancer patients, control medical schools and medical publications.

"Cancer today is probably somewhere around a $90 billion dollar a year industry," he said. " Most of the medical schools are open today because of contributions from major drug companies. Therefore they teach drugs, the selling of drugs."

Government medicine today requires that everyone with the same disease must be treated the same way. That is the world's worst way to practice medicine, Dr. Binzel declares. No two patients are the same.

He cited a California study in which an internist made a 20-year investigation of patients with lung cancer. Many were treated with surgery, chemotherapy and radiation, but a large number chose not to have any treatment at all.

"After following the non-treatment group as closely as he followed the treated group," Dr. Binzel said, "the doctor found that the survival time of those who were treated with surgery, radiation and chemotherapy was three and a half years. The survival time of those who refused any treatment at all was twelve years. His conclusion was we are killing them four times more rapidly than if we did nothing at all."

Dr. Binzel's reaction to the slogan, "The War On Cancer", is that there is no such war. "The war is to prevent anybody from interfering with the way they are treating cancer."

His treatment belief is that if you just remove the tumor and do nothing to correct the condition that allowed the tumor to develop in the first place, that tumor is going to come back. If not in that area, then some place else. But it is going to come back.

Frequently by the time he sees patients they have had all the radiation and chemotherapy they can have, their defense mechanism is badly damaged or destroyed, there is little to work with.

"There is nothing original in this whole nutritional therapy program with me. The only thing I have done, I have read what these men (Krebs, Nieper, Contreras, etc.) wrote, and did what they said we should do. And I found if I did exactly what they said, and how to do it, it works. There is no question it works, if you do it properly. If you get to these people in time."

* * *

Author's note:

I learned of Dr. Binzel by reading his book, "Alive and Well", which was sent to me by a friend after he learned that my wife was suffering from cancer. The fervor and dedication he displayed in his writings made a very deep impression on me. His concern was obviously entirely for the patient and the quality of life.

He was willing to endure, indeed resist with all means available to him, the efforts of Ohio medical professionals in their attempts to discredit him and to remove his license to practice medicine.

Dr. Binzel is now retired but still provides assistance to many people who find themselves suffering from cancer. His dedication to his fellow human beings as well as his concern for the quality of life of those who are suffering has made an indelible impression on me of a person who does not look at people as a laboratory experiment. Nor is he willing to accept a robotic approach to treatment that ignores completely or at least to a great extent, the increased suffering caused by the treatment.

He and Mrs. Binzel, with whom I chatted briefly after our interview with the doctor, are charming, concerned people who understand and look at people as individuals. They are both highly educated, intelligent and are inordinately understanding and concerned.

My life and outlook have been influenced by this great man and the example of sacrifice and endurance he has provided. I am certain that any appreciation I have for his work is far exceeded by those whose suffering has been treated and whose lives have been extended.

Dr. Binzel epitomizes my new found understanding of the need to maintain a quality of life rather that to spend our final days in pain, nausea and suffering.

* * *

CHAPTER TWELVE

Interview with:
   Dr. Sandra M. Stewart-Pinkham, M.D.
   General Practitioner
   Columbus, Ohio

Dr. Sandra M. Stewart-Pinkham considers her cancer patients on a case-by-case basis and keeps an open attitude on treatments.

"I like nutritional therapy because I believe you can use it with chemotherapy, radiation and surgery as a complementary therapy," said the Columbus, Ohio, physician.

Originally a pediatrician and now a general practitioner, she actually considers herself a "Psycho-Neuro-Immuno-Endo-Toxicologist".

Everything is connected, she believes, explaining that all facets of her patients are important - their personality, their diet, whether they take nutrient supplements, and how their endocrine system is working.

"The more we see our life as a gift and responsibility, we understand that it's our responsibility to take into ourselves nourishing food for the body to work," she explained. "In order to realize your life, you must have spiritual food. You have to give meaning to your life, be connected with people, and not be in conflict."

It's important to consider all these aspects of the patient and be "flexible" in recommending treatment, she explained.

"When I have a patient with cancer, I like to get a careful history, because I want them to know and I want to know how did this person get cancer? How did this immune system fail to get rid of this?"

She tracks patients' lives to learn if they had a genetic pre-disposition for cancer, if their diet exposed them to a lot of pesticides, if they drank a lot of alcohol, or if they were subjected to cigarette smoke.

"It's sad," she said, when some patients who are treated with chemotherapy and radiation are not investigated first as to whether they came down with cancer because of dietary factors, if their life was stressful or if there were other causation factors.

The doctor believes chemotherapy and radiation are very helpful in some cases, but she does not recommend it for all patients.

"If it is at least seventy percent sure it is going to cure them, I would suggest chemotherapy for anyone over 65 because the quality of life is so important. Newer treatments like endostatin and shark cartilage which prevent the growth of blood vessels into tumors lack side effects and are more desirable."

Some cancers are sensitive to treatment and there are ways to judge the potential results, such as looking at the metallothionein expression. In breast cancer, for example, if there is not a lot of metallothionein expression, the tumors are sensitive to chemotherapy/radiation. Dr. Stewart-Pinkham said if there is an increase in metallothionein and resistance to cadmium, a metal that accumulates in the body and plays a role in cancer, she would advise against chemotherapy.

"Don't do something that would hurt the patient if you don't have a really good chance of cure," she explained.

The situation can be different for younger people. "Sometimes with chemo/radiation, they are curing young people, so I say fine. But with older people you have so much more toxicity. My feeling is they should be candidates for alternative therapies more quickly," she said.

This is particularly true in "Stage Four" or late-stage disease, she explained. There are not many Stage Four diseases that really respond well to chemo/radiation because usually it will not destroy the last cell.

"If you can't get the last cell, it's just going to come back and get worse," she said. "That's why I like to use the alternative approaches for older patients."

"My belief is that older people may suffer more bad effects because their tissue isn't as hardy to begin with and the quality of life to me is especially critical," Dr. Stewart-Pinkham said. "A lot of younger people are willing to suffer through chemo/radiation because they feel it will save their lives, and if it does save their lives, sure it's worthwhile."

The doctor says she agrees with recommendations of the Cancer Treatment Centers of America. Patients given nutritional therapy, or good nutrition, are more able to tolerate chemotherapy and radiation is improved.

"I say to people I can't tell you what you should do. Besides, I can't cure your cancer. It's your body that will do that, if it can. But I can advise you on how to use nutrition."

Part of Dr. Stewart-Pinkham's approach to cancer treatment and nutritional therapy involves her great interest in the role cadmium may play in the body with its both helpful and harmful effects. Cadmium in animal studies has been shown to act as an anti-carcinogen to fight cancer at high doses, and in low doses can be a carcinogen by increasing the resistance of cancer cells to current treatments.

She urges a great deal more research on how cadmium may be an important connection between health and the environment.

She feels our current investigative models are inadequate for understanding how very low concentrations of chemicals like cadmium or electromagnetic fields can produce disruptions, affecting reproduction and development, and causing malformations and cancer.

Cadmium first interested Dr. Stewart-Pinkham a decade ago when she was a pediatrician working with children with learning disabilities. She conducted a study using hair and learned that lead and cadmium levels in hair were elevated in youngsters who had poor scores on achievement tests.

"It seemed to me that heavy metals that were occurring at very low doses were having some toxic effects which were affecting the brain functions of children," she said.

She learned from a biochemist that lead probably would not have caused the effects but that cadmium was highly toxic. The question was raised about what caused the exposure.

She learned that cadmium is an ubiquitous pollutant, meaning it is found virtually everywhere, but the most important source to humans is active and passive cigarette smoke. Another factor in the community where Dr. Pinkham practiced medicine was a trash-burning power plant that emitted a ton of cadmium every year for 10 years. It was closed in 1994.

As she learned about cadmium, she found it could be the chemical connection influencing how stress could cause various effects such as heart disease, cancer, degenerative diseases and auto-immune diseases.

She considered the possibility that emotional stress mobilizes free cadmium in the body. Cadmium can interact with other chemicals to affect the cell membrane, interfere with DNA repair, and impair mitrocardial functions, so that the host cell is more susceptible to cancer.

"The paradox is that here, a carcinogenic agent that functions also as a co-carcinogen can also be an anti-carcinogen," she said. "I think cadmium is so interesting because it has so many abilities to affect so many facets of cells. I would encourage researchers in any particular problem to include studying the effects of cadmium on that problem because of its ability to effect so many processes".

She believes that when chemotherapy and radiation are used to kill cancer cells, they are effective partly because cadmium is released and plays some role in destroying the cancer.

"The trouble is the cadmium causes so much injury to everything else - the liver, kidney, the brain, blood vessels and the endocrine system," she explained. "If we had some way of selectively killing the cancer, that would be better."

Cadmium also could be operating in viral infections such as HIV infection and influenza. It can cause mutations, and has a tremendous ability to bind to various molecules that have a function in cells, she explained.

People are born with very little cadmium in their bodies, unless their mothers smoked cigarettes. But organs such as the liver continue to accumulate it during a lifetime. The kidney, which has a lot of cadmium, accumulates it until about the age 50, then it decreases.

"My feeling is that as you lose your ability to make good proteins, which happens with aging, then you have more free cadmium. Then free cadmium, because of its ability to cause oxidized stress, can then promote these effects of aging, such as cancer," stated Dr. Steward-Pinkham as she continued her firm belief in the role that Cadmium may play.

The doctor's interest in nutritional therapy began before she treated cancer patients, but worked with women who complained of feeling tired. Both groups had the same symptoms, she later learned.

"A lot of those who came in were tired and weak. They felt bad. I think that can happen for a variety of reasons. A lot of women with cancer are over tired, have pushed themselves too long, worked too hard, and haven't rested enough," she s aid. "They are worn down. That is part of getting cancer, not having enough energy in your immune system to get rid of it."

When they are given nutrients to kill off fungus, given essential fatty acids to help their mitochondria produce energy in the cells, they recover and feel better, she said.

"The quality of life comes back, even though they may not be curing themselves of the disease. I'm always trying to improve the quality of life," she explained.

The doctor has experienced success with patients in nutritional therapy.

• The most prominent case involved a Columbus woman who had breast cancer. Her heart was enlarged, which was a contraindication for chemotherapy and radiation, so she turned to alternative therapy as her only option. The patient had tumor cells which had spread to her bone marrow.

The 41-year-old patient began a fish and vegetable diet, ate organic food, took vitamins, nutrient-rich foods, and supplements such as Coenzyme Q 10. She began an exercise program. Dr. Pinkham referred her to the book, "You Can't Afford The Luxury of a Single Negative Thought."

Within a month, her tumor markers were down, and today are undetectable. She has no evidence of the disease.

• Another female patient declined to have chemotherapy or radiation for her metastatic ovarian cancer. She had partial surgery. She was an herbalist and began a vegetarian diet. She quit her job and stayed home because as Dr. Pinkham said, "her job was to get rid of cancer." Her tumor markers went down in six weeks and have never come back up again.

• One woman with metastatic ovarian cancer clearly improved with nutritional therapy.

• Another patient with metastatic disease to the hip experienced a decrease in pain and felt better.

"My own approach is that the patient comes first, and if the patient benefits from this alternative therapy, then it's worth it. I find they are benefiting," she said.

At the same time, Dr. Stewart-Pinkham feels she differs from other physicians on this opinion.

"There are so few, it's sad," she said. "The medical school here doesn't have any interest in it. The attitude of the average doctor is they don't know and don't really want to become involved because there is

76

some kind of feeling of quackery. Some of them are very outspoken and very hostile to anybody who uses it."

There has been criticism in the medical profession that such therapies are not supported by studies or trials. Dr. Pinkham believes "the trial is the person. My role is to help the person."

She informs patients she can not know the response they will have from anything she recommends for them, but their response will tell them whether it is working.

"To me, what is important is how the individual responds, so it doesn't matter if there is no study about it. I feel I have studied cadmium. I know a lot about the biochemistry. I know a lot about how it can work and how the body can help itself. You don't try to say ahead of time - well, this is going to work, because there are so many variables. You can't do that kind of trial. Besides everybody is unique. Even if there was some trial, this person may not respond anyway," she said.

Dr. Stewart-Pinkham believes that stresses can be a factor in cancer, but they are hard to avoid in the average life. That's why she recommends the book about not having a negative thought.

"You can't afford it if you have cancer, and you can't afford it if you don't want to get cancer, she said. "That's why I'm interested in stress."

She had one female patient with breast cancer whose husband had testicular cancer. They were farmers and exposed to pesticides, but their daughter had died of an accidental choking in their barn three years before they got the cancer.

She stated that, "I highly respect the power of severe stress, which can be whatever is stressful for the individual such as a loss of a loved one, a divorce or a betrayal by a business partner".

"If patients are in knots about something, it starts eating away at them," she said. "I noticed in my studies of people with cancer, there were different stresses for different people. But many times, five to ten years before the cancer occurred, there were very painful things that happened."

The stress of caring for people with cancer could even trigger the disease in the caretaker. What could happen in such cases is that chronic stress could cause the release of cadmium and it becomes destructive when not detoxified.

Once a person has cancer, she is convinced some oncologists proceed with chemotherapy and radiation with only a slight chance of recovery because they feel not to do it would be to abandon the patient, not give them any hope.

She believes if a patient does not have a good prognosis of responding to those treatments, they shouldn't be given, especially if it's an older patient. Instead, she suggests alternative nutritional therapy and supporting the immune system.

"You're not dead until you're dead. So if every day of your life is a high-quality day, you have plenty of energy, and you can make the most of your life, that's the way to do it," she said.

It's sometimes important to discuss death with patients, she believes, to inform them what forms death can take and to make them appreciate having lived a rewarding life.

"Everybody dies. We all die," she said. " I say, your life has been a blessing to all these people, you've lived a good life, what do you have to fear of dying? So I would say, Go for it! Fight the cancer, but by improving the quality of life, if the cancer progresses, well, this is not a bad death. You get to say good-bye."

Dr. Stewart-Pinkham generally shares with her cancer patients that their disease is a wake-up call for them to change their lifestyles because what they were doing allowed the cancer to develop.

"If you want to help yourself while you're going through treatment," she tells them, "eat really good food, have this happiness to forgive and forget, let the past be past, and enjoy life."

* * *

Author's Note:

The interview with Dr. Stewart-Pinkham revealed a woman who is both a medical doctor and a person full of compassion and concern for the quality of life a patient may experience. She is one of a growing number of physicians becoming aware that treatment often can be worse than the disease.

Medical doctors are commendable who ask questions, consider quality of life of the patient and are willing to risk the consequences of the certain criticism from some who practice only conventional medicine.

Doctors like Dr. Stewart- Pinkham, in their effort to maintain a quality of life, especially for older patients, deserve the thanks of all who could be spared the pain and agony of conventional treatment in a hopeless procedure.

Dr. Stewart-Pinkham has helped me overcome some of the overwhelming depression I felt after realizing the hopelessness of conventional treatment in certain situations. Learning about an alternative which can maintain some degree of life quality, self respect and hope can be a shining ray for many who dwell in the darkness of despair.

History will remember these people who dared go beyond what is conventionally accepted. I hope knowing of my personal gratitude, as well as that of her patients, will make her work a little easier.

* * *

CHAPTER THIRTEEN

Searching for Possible Cures

This book is for those people who find themselves dealing with a specific type of cancer: Metastasized Small- Cell Lung Cancer. It may also be a source of information for other patients or caregivers, confused and distressed by what they are hearing from the medical profession, who may be wondering if there are better answers.

There are a number of unconventional or alternative treatments to surgery, chemotherapy and radiation, with some touted as cures or accused as quackery. A few that are better known and claim success are shark cartilage, flaxseed oil, special extractions from natural substances such as Cat's Claw, DHEA, Laetrile, and special nutritional approaches based upon what is called "microbiotics".

I am not taking a position one way or the other on any of the non-traditional cancer procedures, but I wish I had been given more time to investigate them before my wife's death after chemotherapy and radiation therapy only intensified her agony.

The beliefs I share in this chapter are a result of personal observation of what my wife went through, in combination with many hours of reading and researching questions.

I found very little documented or accepted results with respect to non-conventional treatment for the type of cancer she suffered. The horrible effects of standard practice are known to me first hand.

When Meryl's cancer was originally diagnosed, we were told rather bluntly that no surgery was indicated and that nothing could be done about the lung cancer. Little more was said other than a biopsy was needed to determine what kind of cancer she had. What we were told in effect amounted to nothing more than a death warrant.

Once the shock had worn off, we felt we had to look for other answers. Her best friend told us of a clinic in Oklahoma and said she would attempt to make contact. This was not successful but another clinic was found in El Paso with the actual facility located in Juarez, Mexico. This launched our first experience in trying to improve her odds of survival.

We began her fight against cancer with a commitment to go to the clinic. The decision was made out of desperation and total ignorance. Yet, this was the beginning of a search on my part to find as much information on metastisized small-cell lung cancer as possible.

I have always been a person with an insatiable curiosity, a thirst for knowledge that has grown over the years. Accepting conditions without asking "WHY" is a position I have always rejected.

As I became more and more familiar with many doctors and hospitals, I began to realize that any references to unconventional treatments often were blocked with open hostility. A certainty that became painfully evident to me early on was the huge amount of disdain and even hate that exists between the medical profession and doctors who delve into non-conventional treatment.

For the most part, doctors who practice conventional medicine do not seem interested in anything other than what is conventional. Yet, many doctors who are mailing out newsletters make strong cases for supplements and alternative treatment.

Medical education is very intensive and detailed, undoubtedly leaving doctors little time to consider anything other than tools and information necessary to conduct their standard procedures. However, progress comes when someone goes beyond what is known and searches for the unknown. Those who merely practice what they know without a curiosity, will never learn more. It's similar to my father's old saying, "If we only talk and never listen, then we are limited to what we already know".

Those who go beyond the known are those who are never satisfied with answers and never stop asking questions, both of themselves and the outside world. Individuals can never move ahead unless they ask "why" each time they find that what is known is not enough.

Dedication to accepted treatment methods, even when it is known that the results are totally unacceptable, will rarely result in improvement. It is this fact of blind acceptance, coupled with the fanatic criticism of those who dare challenge the status quo, that may be the greatest deterrent to finding a cure for cancer or at least, meaningful progress.

Acceptance of having nothing more available than surgery, radiation and chemotherapy leaves me with a greatly reduced appreciation of some aspects of the medical profession.

I have to wonder if there could be some improvement in treatment results if more cooperation existed within the medical profession. Otherwise, it may continue its status quo.

A surgeon stated in one book I read that he successfully performed hundreds of surgical procedures in his lifetime. He felt that at the end of his career he had not contributed anything to the progress of medicine. The doctor was well aware he performed competently what he knew and had been taught. But he improved on nothing except perhaps his own dexterity. Yet, in this era of fault finding, the fear of malpractice and litigation obviously are important reasons to discouraging personal initiative.

The claims of great progress about which we read everyday are to some degree true. But for the most part, even though there has been some improvement in drugs, and development of new drugs such as Epogen and Neupogen, certain types of cancer still are short-time death warrants. During the course of treatment, the cost in quality of life to me is totally unacceptable. The cost in dollars is beyond comprehension.

It was interesting and dismaying to me that the cost of conventional treatment always seemed to be justified. Yet, procedures outside those traditionally accepted were considered terribly expensive. One doctor who became rather candid with me stated that conventional treatment usually is covered by insurance and thus is not a recognized expense.

Alternatives normally are not covered by insurance and therefore are more costly. I find this to be rather interesting logic and a poor excuse in the fight against anything non-conventional.

This doctor also remarked that if a cure for lung cancer were to be found or people would stop smoking, an entire wing of the hospital would have to close, many people would be out of work and the companies who provide cancer drugs would suffer terrible losses. I do not believe it was intended to mean anything other than what a terrible impact cancer has on society and our economy. I discussed this aspect with many people. Only the caring doctors seemed to understand.

I could not help but consider that with all the great progress our society has made in every aspect of science, medicine and engineering, that we have failed miserably in the overall fight against cancer and particularly certain cancers. But a terrible thought which continues to haunt me is the one the doctor placed in my mind predicting the great economic disaster if a cure were found.

A multi-billion dollar industry exists based on the current status quo of killer cancers. The economic result of a cure would be devastating for some elements of our society. I learned there are many others like me who wonder at times if there are some in our society who really want to find a cure. But many are paying for their livelihood

From my limited exposure to the approach in finding answers, the rules seem to discourage an acceleration of the search.

Certainly, some prevailing attitudes do raise suspicions in many people's minds.

Ironically, it seems some doctors who treat cancer become willing candidates for alternative treatment themselves if they personally have developed the dreaded killer. Who could be a better endorsement for the currently accepted treatments than doctors who perform the procedures? What could be more of an indictment than a doctors' unwillingness to accept standard procedures for themselves?

A number of doctors today are becoming more and more convinced the conventional approach as we know it is nothing more than the poisoning and destruction of the body. The majority however, still maintain that the trio of surgery, radiation and chemotherapy is this generation's answer to cancer.

Many medical professionals who operate non-conventional treatment centers find it necessary to locate them outside the United States. Those who practice within our borders quite often do so at great risk of being able to continue their careers.

One Texas physician who claims to have found a cure has been under constant attack. The medical profession, the Federal Drug Administration and others have been trying for sometime to discredit him and revoke his license to practice medicine.

Doctor Stanislaw Brezynski, a Polish native came to this country several years ago. He was seeking freedom to pursue his beliefs and research in finding a cure for cancer.

He opened a clinic in Houston, Texas, where he has developed a non-toxic drug and named it "Antineoplaston". While he has been able to continue his work, he has been under constant attacks by the Federal Drug Administration and Attorney General's office. Until now, only

83

favorable court decisions, have saved him from total discredit. Doctors and certainly many of his patients have come to his assistance by testifying and raising money to help pay his legal costs.

At this writing he has again been acquitted, and the FDA is supporting tests on his procedures.

From the time of my wife's cancer diagnosis, I began reading and researching everything I could find about cancer. It's interesting that once a person responds to a mailing about any subject, from that time on, the volume of mail becomes almost overwhelming.

I began receiving flyers from many who either claimed to be experts in medicine or were individuals with PhD's in some health field. Most were from doctors soliciting subscriptions to their medical news letters.

It became obvious very quickly that the strength of their appeals for subscriptions was in pointing out the dangers of conventional medical treatment. The statement,

"What your doctor won't tell you," or a paraphrase was used to convince those who received this information that the medical profession was totally oblivious to anything outside the usual practice of, "see the doctor and get a prescription". In fact, after reading flyer after flyer, every advertisement was directed toward a conviction that the medical profession including doctors, drugs and hospitals were bad for one's health. Even statements like, "What you don't know could kill you", were not uncommon.

While most of the medical news letters were written by doctors, or those who claimed to be, they were characterized by comments proclaiming better ways to treat illnesses than prescription drugs. Also, and in almost every case, the reader was cautioned that surgery as a cure was usually not necessary.

The theme contained in most flyers and descriptive material was generally the same. They stated or inferred that too many doctors lacked knowledge about non-conventional treatments being used successfully.

The literature claimed alternative methods were available for everything from cancer to high blood pressure, arthritis, disease of the liver and kidneys, skin problems, indigestion, vision, hearing, prostate and many others. If a medical problem exists, the documents alleged, there is a supplement, herb, vitamin and/or exercise that will be a better solution than risking the effects of prescription drugs or surgery.

For example, a herb called Bilberry is recommended for eye problems: Echinacea is touted as a natural anti-biotic; Cayenne powder is advertised to reduce high blood pressure without serious side effects or the impotence occurring in men who take prescription drugs.

When a person is desperate and faces certain death, as certainly is the case with metastisized small-cell lung cancer, with little time available, any idea proposed by supposedly knowledgeable people is welcome.

Most who face the terrible dilemma of a short-term, terminal cancer or other illness want to find a cure, inside or outside conventional medicine. Some desperate people, in their urgency to hold onto life, can be gullible to expensive quackery that only offers illusions. They grasp at anything to stall the prognosis of certain death, or that can only offer a brief delay. The time they are fighting may not be years, but rather months, a few weeks or days.

To make sure that I am not misunderstood, there is no doubt in my mind that most doctors are doing what they have been taught and believe to be the only acceptable methods of treatment. I also am sure that peer pressure, risk of losing the license to practice, fear of malpractice, the threat of litigation and just lack of time are factors in maintaining the status quo.

One positive indicator of lack of time is that patients and/or caretakers such as myself are posing questions and offering information about the newest procedures or medications. Doctors tend to be puzzled as to their source. I found that it surprises medical professionals when lay persons come up with such information. Yet, universities, libraries, doctors who publish and the widening Internet are all sources of information.

Originally, I thought finding literature about small-cell lung cancer, treatments, and others cancers would be difficult and perhaps a near impossibility. I learned a wealth of information was available. Local libraries are accessible to everyone, with an amazing amount of information on both conventional and alternative treatments. People with a personal computer and modem have an inexhaustible supply of data on what is going on throughout the world in cancer research and treatment by accessing the Internet.

The fact that so many doctors are not able to utilize these sources for the most part is that they just do not have the time.

In addition to the traditional medical seminars and training to keep doctors updated, something needs to be done to allow them time for their practices and to keep up on what seems to be an infinite amount of information. The quantity seems to be ever increasing and each day something new is published. Instead of a closed mind to what is new, consideration of the latest, the newest and the potential benefits should be considered.

The world will be far better off as a result. This brings me to several final points. First, I am now convinced there is no cure for the most part for small-cell lung cancer.

Using conventional treatment, once the disease has become entrenched and has spread, the statistics I have read and been told are true, at least in the case of my wife. Survival for most will be 4 to 11 months, with less than 5% experiencing survival to two years.

Next, while there are many claims of cures using alternative treatment, few cases are documented in a manner which is acceptable to the medical profession. They have not been verified with qualified test results, doubters claim.

But my final conclusion is that where there is no cure and the quality of life is being destroyed, being able to live out our remaining days in dignity overrides every other consideration.

* * *

CHAPTER FOURTEEN

Some Claims of Alternative Cancer Cures

Much is being written about all types of cures that are outside the conventional practice of medicine. A variety of literature is available about non-toxic treatments conducted literally all over the world. Information also is available which attempts to explain the causes of cancer.

Yet after my many months of poring over everything I could find on an unbelievable number of approaches to non-conventional cures, one final consideration remained with me.

Documentation to support the claims often either did not exist or was not provided.

While cure claims offered hope of a better quality of life, if nothing else, only a few of the various methods of treatment provided verified information on which a person could make a positive judgment.

I had hoped for more. But any conclusions at which I or anyone else could arrive, in my opinion, would have to be for the most part on the basis of trust rather than facts. However, some of my research did produce some very convincing alternatives.

Looking back now with the experience and knowledge of my wife's terrible experience, the wisdom of hindsight rules.

I have wondered many times, as I mentioned earlier, what might have been if we had stopped the radiation and chemotherapy after the initial improvement and chanced one or more of the alternative treatments available.

If that had failed and her death came about, without a doubt I would have blamed myself for not staying in the conventional mainstream.

Now, I know the terrible truth which is that the few days of feeling better after radiation and chemotherapy was nothing more than the lull before the storm. If I had it to do over, I would not hesitate to try one or more of the various non-conventional treatments. This, of course, would have been with my wife's concurrence.

I have to accept now what I could not at first, that patients with Metastasized Small-Cell Lung Cancer have a life expectancy of four to eleven months, and less than 5% live beyond that to two years. My wife was not totally aware of these statistics.

Convinced of these death-sentence figures which are certain, based on today's conventional treatments, and facing such deadlines, my concern is no longer a matter of life or death, but the quality of life for whatever time remains.

The unproved projection of a few more days or weeks of life with conventional treatment - producing all the attending debilitation, fear, pain and self-esteem destruction such as the loss of hair, is simply morally wrong. But accepting death in a short time belies the human trait of hope.

So, with the wisdom of hindsight, and if I were given the chance to do it over again, I would have stopped the standard procedures. I believe the proper time would have been after the first or second round of chemotherapy. Then as soon as she was well enough to travel, my choice would have been to try something else.

I would no longer have the apprehension of what is wrong and right. Knowing death is certain in the short term negates any feeling of blame. Experiencing alternative treatment, perhaps even shortening life and adding better life quality, would now be my choice. If I personally am diagnosed with cancer, my choice without hesitation would be for alternative treatment. Facing certain death and having to live when the quality of life has been destroyed means struggling to gulp in breaths to live but not breathing the essence of life.

Modern medicine and its treatment of Metastatic Small Cell Lung Cancer is barbaric, cruel, impersonal, expensive and utterly fails to show any sign of humane consideration.

Obviously my attitude has changed from what it was in February when we were told my wife had lung cancer and that it had spread to her spine. This state of mind partly evolved from investigating some of the following alternative treatments my wife may have tried if we had been given the time.

Listed below are some of the many non-conventional methods that have been and are being tried. Keep in mind, however, there is little or no documentation available on any procedure which conventional medicine seems not willing to accept or consider.

SHARK CARTILAGE:

People interested in this approach to a cancer cure will find a number of publications available. I read two books written by Dr. I. William Lane regarding his research and effort in the use of shark cartilage. His first book was entitled, "Sharks Don't Get Cancer". A follow-up is called, "Sharks Still Don't Get Cancer" (Avery Publishing, $12.95).

The publication provides information on the qualities of the processed cartilage as well as dosages which have been tried. The doctor claims the success rate on tumor remission has been astounding.

Shark cartilage is available from all health stores and nutrition agencies. The use and dosage is detailed to some extent in Dr. Lane's books.

Some mainstream medical authorities have branded Dr. Lane a "quack", according to Dennis Fiely, a reporter for Accent. In a November, 1996 article, he reported that the Food and Drug Administration has approved the beginning of "the first human clinical trials. These trials are to test the effect of shark cartilage on tumor growth."

FLAXSEED OIL

A number of individuals have experimented with flaxseed oil in treating various diseases. I was impressed with what I have read about the work of Dr. Johanna Budwig, a German Nobel Prize nominee. Highly respected as Germany's premier biochemist, Dr. Budwig has published several books including "Cancer - A Fat Problem" and "The Death of The Tumor".

Dr. Budwig has treated seriously ill cancer patients with flaxseed oil and low fat cottage cheese. According to her reports, over a period of approximately three months, tumors gradually receded. Symptoms of cancer, liver dysfunction, anemia and diabetes were completely alleviated.

According to a book written by Ingeborg M. Johnston, C.N., and James R. Johnston, Ph.D., entitled Flaxseed Oil and the Power of Omega-3, Dr. Budwig reported in 1953 that she could change the yellow-green protein substance in the blood to healthy red blood pigment or hemoglobin by giving cancer patients four ounces of non fat cottage cheese and three tablespoons of fresh flax oil each day for three months. She also reported that lipoproteins and phosphtides, previously lacking, reappeared.

If effective as alleged, the results possibly could eliminate the need for the drugs Neupogen and Epogen which are used to help restore a patient's blood levels after chemotherapy treatments. Even though these two drugs have proven to be very successful, the cost over a period of several months could run into thousands of dollars. For example, Neupogen costs nearly $140 per vial. Ten injections were prescribed after each chemo treatment, which in my wife's case was every four weeks.

LAETRILE AND OTHER NUTRITIONAL THERAPIES;

Dr. Philip E. Binzel, Jr., M.D., whose interview is included in this book, began to investigate the role of nutrition in human disorders in 1974 after becoming a General Practitioner in Washington Court House, Ohio, in 1955.

According to his book, "Alive and Well", published in 1994 by American Media, he has a record of astounding success in treating cancer patients. He documents by name a number of patients who did not expect to survive their cancer, many of whom are still alive and well today.

I talked with him personally about treating my wife but by the time I was able to make contact, she was only two days from her death and unable to leave her bed. Thus, another possible alternative was not explored. Her confidence in her oncologist and her perceived improvement in her condition kept me in a mental state of being terribly uncertain about what to do.

Laetrile is a substance made from apricot pits. There have been statements made by the medical community that it is a poison and contains Hydrogen Cyanide, thus making it toxic. It appears to have been proven that Laetrile itself does not contain Cyanide, but rather causes it to be released in the presence of cancer cells.

Dr. Binzel uses Laetrile both orally and intravenously along with a certain approved diet that includes whole grains, corn, butter, nuts, buckwheat, dried fruit and beans. Beverages are restricted. Milk is limited to cereals and cooking. Caffeine is not permitted.

DHEA - DEHYDROEPIANDROSTERONE:

DHEA is a brain nutrient and has been available as a prescription drug for some time. It is a naturally occurring phospholipid nutrient, a steroid hormone produced by the adrenal glands. In recent months, it has been released for over the counter purchase and it can be obtained without a prescription.

According to Health Watchers System, Arthur Schwartz, a biochemist at Temple University, administered DHEA to mice and observed an incredible reversal of aging: old mice regained youthful vigor. Cancer, whether naturally occurring or induced by artificial means, disappeared. Immune response increased, life span increased by 20%.

It is claimed that forty thousand medical studies and articles regarding DHEA have shown that low DHEA levels in humans correlate to increased risk of cancer, heart disease, osteoporosis, obesity, diabetes and premature aging. In America, 83% of all deaths are from cancer and heart disease.

As the information about DHEA has spread, it has become one of the fastest selling, nonprescription supplements on the market. How DHEA will affect those who are now using it is unknown. But a number of articles have been published cautioning that its use should be restricted. Most of what I have read states that men should not exceed dosages of 50 to 100 milligrams daily and women should use half as much, perhaps 25 to 50 milligrams.

CAT'S CLAW (UNO DE GATO)

Cat's Claw was first brought to my attention in Mexico where my wife was treated initially. It comes from South America and was recommended by one of the doctors on the staff of the clinic. It is alleged to cause cancerous tumors to shrink.

It can be obtained in most places that sell supplements. There is a great variation in price and quality, which requires careful shopping by users.

According to the staff doctor mentioned, it is to be taken before each meal. The recommended quantity was three capsules before each meal. We purchased a supply upon our return home and used it for several months. It was stopped after she no longer wanted to take anything, not even her prescription drugs.

MICROBIOTICS:

Numerous articles and books have endorsed the importance of diets in the treatment of cancer. Books have been written by doctors who contracted cancer and who knew what to expect with conventional treatment. Fellow doctors were horrified that the cancer victim refused conventional treatment and urged their reconsideration. In each case, the doctors who were able to conquer cancer attributed their victories to the diets they adopted.

The information is easily available in libraries and other sources. The diet approach involves the elimination of fats. Foods such as brown rice and seaweed are important elements, and red meat is not allowed during the early portion of the diet.

Dr. Binzel, to whom I referred earlier, used the microbiotics approach along with Laetrile. When I interviewed him, he said he provided the details and education to patients, but it was up to them to carry it out.

TEA - GREEN AND HORSETAIL:

Among the many proposed cancer fighters and immune system builders are various kinds of tea. The one most mentioned is Green Tea. Some authors believe the incidence of cancer is lower in Japan because the population drinks a great deal of Green Tea. I have not found any clinical trials or available data which proves that green tea has any real effect. Most of what I have read or heard is without any positive backing, facts or tests.

Horsetail Tea or as it is called in Mexico, Te de Cola de Cabola, is recommended by many doctors south of the border as a cancer fighter. It is not especially delightful to drink but as with any hot beverage, the taste is secondary to the benefits. The one thing my wife enjoyed every morning during her illness, until she could no longer tolerate food or drink, was a hot cup of tea. That was her standard order the first thing every morning, even before I was able to start preparing breakfast.

Tap water is another item that should be mentioned. A chiropractor once told her not to drink tap water but to start using **bottled or purified water**. I purchased a container which held two gallons of water. For cooking and drinking, I used nothing else. If our water contains contaminants of the scale that we are being told, I felt this was necessary. However, I am also aware that when water is purified, all the minerals are also removed which eliminates water as a primary source of such minerals as sodium, calcium, magnesium, potassium, iron and others. As a result, supplements take on even more importance.

Removing such items as chlorine and other impurities from the water, however, seems to be considered absolutely necessary.

MISCELLANEOUS OTHER HOME REMEDIES:

There are many more supplements advertised that fight cancer, boost the immune system and in general, tone the body to conduct its own fight against disease.

These include vitamins, herbs, minerals, etc. Anything that helps build normal body functions, improves the immune system, builds resistance, helps the liver, kidneys, heart, and other organs are favored to help the body fight disease. While chemotherapy can kill cancer cells, it also is devastating to the immune system, blood, kidneys and liver. At some time during chemotherapy treatment, according to the makers of Neupogen and Epogen, vital functions will begin to fail so that required signals to keep bodily functions at normal levels will cease. These two expensive prescription drugs are used to provide what kidneys and liver can no longer do in restoring normal blood levels.

Vitamins ranging from A through Z, herbs of all sorts with names that carry no familiarity and minerals such as iron, copper, magnesium, calcium, are all stated to be necessary for the body and its immune system to function normally. For example, bone allegedly will deteriorate and look like Swiss Cheese if sufficient calcium is not absorbed. Literature also states certain kinds of calcium are absorbed better than others, and magnesium is necessary in the process.

There are huge amounts of material available. These include written, audio and video. As an example, there is a book written by James F. Balch, M.D. and Phyllis A. Balch, C.N.C., entitled "Prescription for Nutritional Healing".

I scoured every source I could find, perused various publications and brought home only those which I felt addressed our needs. The number of cancer fighters goes on and on. I have only shown a few of the most obvious that can be used at home. Even Laetrile is available upon demand by the patient. The law states that a patient cannot be denied access to Laetrile if the patient demands it.

Other possible alternative treatments tend to be restricted to administration at clinics and by qualified attendants, even though many are labeled "quacks" by the medical profession.

Many approaches exist. Treatments range from raising body temperature, to use of interferon, and drawing and treating the patient's blood outside the body with a virus and re-injecting it. Other named treatments include Hoxey, Gersten, Cone, Hydrazine Sulfate, Hydrogen Peroxide, Burzynski's Antineoplastons and on and on.

Some of these will be mentioned later in this book.

* * *

CHAPTER FIFTEEN

Some Facilities Providing Alternative Treatment

After my wife's diagnosis of cancer, we became aware that facilities existed both in the United States and abroad which provided treatment for many different types of disease. These facilities, as a general procedure of practice, did not utilize the conventional treatments of surgery, chemotherapy and radiation that were favored by the medical profession.

However, some of the clinics I have visited provided these procedures if they were deemed appropriate in conjunction with their normal alternative treatments.

I had heard numerous stories over the years about the experiences of patients that had gone to Mexico for treatment. Most of the cases involved the use of Laetrile. Other than that, I knew very little because I had no reason to investigate such facilities. We neither knew the names of such clinics nor did we know specific locations.

While some of the stories seemed almost unbelievable in their alleged cures, I had to wonder that if such a treatment were effective, certainly the medical establishment would be using it in the United States. As time went by and we talked with doctors, nurses and other medical professionals, we learned that most of them were involved in conventional methods and knew little or nothing about these places.

Even with no knowledge, opinions were quite definite. These clinics, according to some of the doctors with whom I conversed, involved quacks and frauds. They quickly pointed out the clinics were very expensive.

When we learned of Meryl's illness, some friends investigated places of alternative treatment and convinced her we should leave immediately for a clinic in Juarez, Mexico. She was to stay two to four weeks, at a cost of $3,500 a week. I thought this was expensive until I got the first hospital bill after we returned home. For a twelve day stay, the total hospital bill came to almost $30,000.

As we delved more and more into unconventional treatment and watched the effects of standard procedures, it was becoming obvious that the latter offered little or no hope for my wife's type of cancer. And so, the search and investigation began into an answer somewhere else.

The more I learned about unconventional procedures, the more I became interested in looking at as many methods as I could possibly find. As my decision to write this book came about, I also determined that I would visit as many of these clinics as I could to find out firsthand what they were doing.

After my wife's death, and after I had written most of the book except for this portion, I began visiting clinics and interviewing doctors. It is important to note that every facility I visited was staffed and operated by medical doctors. My interviews and comments only involve some I visited personally. The only exceptions are two clinics located in the United States which received publicity in the media. My interest in them came primarily from the enthusiastic support they obviously had from their patients.

My first visit was to San Diego, California, where I went to clinics both in that city and Tijuana, Mexico.

* * *

INTERVIEW AT AMERICAN BIOLOGICS HOSPITAL, TIJUANA, MEXICO

An appointment was made the morning after my arrival in San Diego. I registered in The International Motor Inn, a motel less than a mile from the Mexican border in San Ysidro, California. It was recommended by the American Biologics Hospital and most of their ambulant patients stayed there.

Some rooms were equipped with kitchen facilities for those who wanted to do part of their own cooking. I learned later that many out-patients of the Oasis Hospital also stayed there.

The coordinator of the Alivizatos Treatment at The American Biologics Hospital is Kathleen Jewett, a very cordial and charming young lady. She made all the arrangements for the tour of the facilities. The hospital itself is coordinated by Mr. Juan Aguilar and is under the medical direction of Dr. Rodrigo Rodriguez, M.D.

American Biologics utilizes a treatment developed by Dr. Hariton Alivizatos, M.D., PhD, who is a native of Greece. He is a medical doctor and has a doctorate in microbiology.

Mr. Eldon Jewett met Dr. Alivizatos in Greece in November, 1977, where his wife, Peggy, was under treatment by the doctor.

In December, 1983, Mr. Jewett was able to convince Dr. Alivizatos to bring his treatment to the American continent. The doctor returned to his homeland and unfortunately died in his sleep in the spring of 1991. The treatment however, has been continued at American Biologics.

I left the motel the morning of my appointment and traveled on one of the vans which transports patients to the hospital.

When I arrived, several patients were having breakfast in the dining room. I was given permission to chat with patients while they were eating.

By coincidence, I sat down at a table where Mr. Eldon Jewett and his wife, Peggy, were already sitting. He described, during our conversation, how he brought Dr. Alivizatos to Tijuana and established the American Biologics Hospital.

Mr. Jewett talked freely about the origin of the hospital and the various kinds of treatment the hospital provided. I mentioned that my wife and I had been to a clinic in Juarez where their treatment was based primarily on Laetrile, live cell injection and chelation.

I questioned him about live cell and whether it comes from cattle. His response was no, it comes from sheep. He stated that in Romania and Switzerland, they have specialists who do this treatment.

In response to my questions about treatments at the center, he said all items used are natural ingredients found in the human cell.

The human cell consists of 429 ingredients, while the center utilizes 53 ingredients. All of the items in the Alivizatos (Greek) treatment are in the living part of the cell. When the ingredients are combined in a specific manner for the Alivizatos Treatment, they then become a separate entity.

The purpose of one of the ingredients is to open the veins, the arteries and the capillaries so that the treatment can flow through. If the treatment does not get to the cancer, it can not be effective.

Mr. Jewett said he does not have cancer but experienced a lot of surgery from injuries in World War II. He has a lot of internal scar tissue and the treatment goes to where there is an abnormality.

He stated, "Now I say that I don't have cancer - I do have cancer - I have probably ten cancers. You probably have ten. We all do.

"Our immune systems control it, He continued. "Your immune system is doing this when you get colds, when you get the flu, when you get all kinds of things. When the immune system is not working like it should, we get things like arthritis and diabetes, which is the case with my sister."

Treatment, Mr.Jewett explained, is designed to take away the cancer's food, causing the cancer cells to starve and, at the same time, modulating the immune system. If the immune system were strong, people would never have cancer or need treatment. He said the most marvelous system that the Lord ever gave us was the immune system. And people spend their entire lives trying to tear it down.

Mr. Jewett then related the history and background of Dr. Hariton Alivizatos, M.D., PhD., who spent twenty six years in cancer research. Although he was graduated from medical school, he did not pursue his internship. He returned to school and obtained a doctorate in micro-biology. He followed this course because the university in Athens was connected with the large hospital, St. Leo's, which has access to cadavers of Greek people who died of cancer and other diseases.

The doctor was hated in Greece, Mr. Jewett explained, because a Greek official owned major cancer clinics in that country. Alivizatos was gaining a reputation for curing people, actually healing people and taking business away from the Greek official's establishments. Another dignitary later owned cancer clinics, and had a similar reason to oppose Dr. Alivizatos, Mr. Jewett said.

So politics in Greece made it very difficult for Dr. Alivizatos to treat people, even those who had terminal disease. Yet people were coming from all over the world, including the United States, for his treatment.

Mr. Jewett, who during World War II served in the U.S. Navy in the Pacific Theater under Admiral William F. (Bull) Halsey and with Admiral Chester Nimitz's staff, was familiar with personal injury and the deaths of others.

He described his family's experience with his mother-in-law's death. If the family dog had been "10% as ill as she was", he would have put the dog out of its misery, he said.

"They strung this out with her for eight months with chemotherapy and she got so sick, the loss of her hair and nausea. She was a lovely women, 61 years old, and they took everything away from her," he recalled.

"The quality of life is more important than living. In her particular case, after she died, her doctor came to the funeral. When he tried to tell me about it, I said that I think you're a criminal and I don't think you ought to practice medicine."

But in the United States, Mr. Jewett added, conventional medicine only had three things, "they cut, they burn and they poison." Stating he read in the newspaper that cancer deaths are down, he remarked, "Cancer deaths are down because of alternative treatment."

Many alternative treatments are "underground" in the United States, he declared.

"Lots and lots of things are happening. People are not accepting what a doctor says. I went to an ophthalmologist five years ago and he said I was so lucky that I went to him in time. He said I had glaucoma and gave me some medication. I walked out, got on an airplane, came down here, went to our ophthalmologist and she says, `You don't have glaucoma. You're a little high in pressure.' So I went back to my own optometrist to whom I had been going to for 25 years and I said, `What about this?'. He said,`Ah, you don't have glaucoma. Your pressure is a little high. I've got people even higher. It's whatever is normal for the person.'

"But he sent me to see a Washington University School of Medicine doctor who is probably the greatest glaucoma doctor in the United States. He said, `Let me look at you every four months. I don't think you have glaucoma.' That was five years ago. Now he sees me every six months and it's a social thing.

"I don't have to believe what a doctor tells me," Mr. Jewett said. "I subscribe to several publications, I look at medication, I listen when a doctor says you should take this, and I look at it. Then, I look at the contra-indications to it and I say, I don't need this. Why would I subject my body to these contra- indications? Nobody is going to tell me to do something harmful to my body. I went to a cardiologist because down here, these guys run treadmills and what have you once a year. I'm 72 years old and I should take care of myself better than I do. It's interesting how things come out as being very good and two or three years later, it comes out being harmful. How does it get out in the first place?"

I asked Mr. Jewett if he could provide some statistics on treatments. The success ratio on the Alivizatos treatment is about 80%, which covers the quantity of life and the quality of life, he said.

"Now nobody has a contract with the Lord," he continued, "but if you come here, you are very ill, you are given three months to live in deep pain and if all of a sudden, you have no pain and you live three years instead of three months, to us, that is a success. We see miracles every day."

Mr. Jewett cited as an example a woman sitting at the table with us, his cousin's wife.

"She is absolutely a miracle. The doctors here don't believe it because they've never seen anything like it. She has Rheumatoid Arthritis, the worst kind," he explained. "Her father died after spending twenty-two years in bed, totally immobile. We stopped at their home and she couldn't go to the bathroom by herself, couldn't pick up a washcloth, couldn't even pick up a cup of coffee. I said what are you doing for this. A doctor told her to take aspirin, so I said I had to get her down to the clinic. You can see she is okay, and she has to come back about every eight months. She starts to go downhill after about eight months. It's a very debilitating disease. We have people here who are all miracles."

The hospital has a case load of about fifty patients at a time, he said, and could handle more except for time consuming record keeping. Part of the trouble with patients in the United States is they are very mobile, moving to different locations. different things. In foreign countries, you can control your patients, he said.

"Americans are under so much more stress than the people down here. They hang loose. Dr. Alivizatos, all of us, believe that stress is what triggers cancer, doesn't cause it, just triggers it. We all have the capability of having cancer. Stress just triggers it. There are all kinds of stress. It could be financial, it could be marital, lots of different kinds. We spend time with patients on stress."

Patients only return to the center if they have a need, he said, there are no standard recommendations for repeat visits.

I felt extremely fortunate to have had the direct contact with Mr. Jewett on a chance encounter.

He and his wife left the next day, so there was no further conversation.

Later that same morning, however, I was given a tour of the entire clinic by various members of the staff. I was shown the rooms for in-patients, modern equipment and surgical facilities. In appearance, it was a clean and well maintained facility.

The following is a condensed summary of the tour and some of the explanations about hospital procedures: Cancer patients have sessions from 7 to 9 a.m. Treatment for patients on different programs begin after 9 a.m. The sessions are longer than for cancer patients, lasting until 2 or 3 p.m. Patients are informed about the treatments, what they are supposed to do, how to eat properly, how to cook foods and other information. They receive more information every day.

Mr. Jewett's relative receives treatment for arthritis, including Vitamin C and other items given intravenously. One major object is to stimulate the body's immune system.

Snake venom is used at times with Laetrile in specific cancer patients. One test involved obtaining a drop of blood from the patient's finger, viewing it under the microscope and analyzing it to determine what is happening in the body and what kind of treatment is needed.

American Biologics has been treating both in and out-patients in its 20-year history. In-patients obviously receive more attention. The standard cancer treatment continues for 21 days, while 10-day sessions are needed for both arthritis and live-cell programs. The clinic also treats chronic fatigue syndrome, known as fibromialgia, believed caused by a virus.

After one year, some patients return for follow-up treatments from three days to a week.

The center's surgical facilities primarily are for emergency use, since it is not normal procedure to perform surgery initially in treatment. All types of surgery can be performed, however, and chemotherapy and radiation can be part of treatment, if needed and recommended.

Following the clinic tour, some patients questioned what I was doing. They began volunteering information about their personal experiences. I observed an inordinate enthusiasm about what was happening to them. It seemed everyone I encountered wanted to share how their lives had been affected by their decision to come to the clinic.

Included here are some of the comments by patients who seemed overjoyed to be able to talk about what they considered a miraculous recovery.

Patient Interview #1:

John Cunningham, Atlanta, Georgia

"I was on chemo and in stage 5. Then they gave up on me. I came here (ABH). Was hospitalized here for three weeks because I was in a wheel chair and couldn't walk. They had given me so much chemotherapy at home that they had destroyed the nerves in my legs. I had kidney failure, damage to my liver, blood pressure. I hadn't eaten for three months. I was being fed intravenously. They had given up on me in Atlanta.

"It has been three years since I came here for the first time. I am alive and well, and that is what is important. Had I not come here, I would have died there. I feel good, I'm walking."

The patient said the person who referred him had cancer, but not as dramatic.

* * *

Patient #2 A middle-age male patient.

"I came here 5 years ago with cancer. Tumors were both inside and outside of my body. Largest ones were on my neck and shoulder. I had been told that I wouldn't live. I couldn't work and was always in pain and nausea. I've been coming here since and I'm still alive. While the tumors outside have not gone away, they are not as large and don't bother me. Main thing is that at home, I can fish, hunt, work and lead a normal life. There is no pain or nausea and except for the growths that remain, I lead a normal life. Even if I still have cancer, I feel fine and I'm still alive. And if you want proof, I still have my hair."

His statement of pride that he still had his hair emphasized the importance of being able to maintain a quality of life.

* * *

Patient #3   A male patient.

"I was told by doctors at home they could do nothing more for me." The patient said he was in pain and vomiting constantly. A friend who received treatment at the clinic referred him.

"This is my second trip for a check-up," he said. "I feel fine and, after 15 months, I'm still alive. Not only that but I am able to do whatever I want at home. Looking at me, nobody would guess that just a year and a half ago, the doctors back home told me to go home and die."

* * *

Patient #4:   A senior female patient.

"I was brought out here on a stretcher. My lung cancer had spread to other parts of my body including my spine and pressure on the spinal chord was causing terrible pain in my legs so that I couldn't walk. I am 63 years old, had been told I had no chance back home and there was nothing more they could do for me.

"Treatment was started here and I just finished the last one. As you can see, I am walking again, there is no more pain and other than feeling weak, I feel a great deal better. My weight had gone down to where I was just a skeleton. While I've gotten back some weight, you can see how thin my legs are so I have a lot of weight to get back again.

" They tell me that this treatment really begins to be effective thirty days after it is finished. So I'm looking forward to a month from now. By then, I should be back to my proper weight."

She questioned if anyone would believe her story who did not know her before she started the treatment.

* * *

Another Patient

My son Dan contacted this patient by telephone at home in Ohio after learning he had been a patient at the American Biologics Hospital. In response to the question that he had been to the clinic in Tijuana, Mexico, for treatment of lung cancer, he responded that he had gone thorough seventeen rounds of chemotherapy before he decided to go to the clinic.

At the clinic, he spent twenty three days there taking the treatment. Afterwards, he came home with the ability to walk, with increased energy and feeling much better.

All he knew was he could only judge by the results, he said. After being told that his time had come, he is now working everyday, sometimes long hours, feels fine and there is no sign of cancer.

"When I got back, my doctor examined me and wanted to give me two more rounds of chemotherapy. I called the clinic, told them what he said and asked what I should do. They told me that it wouldn't hurt and to go ahead. After that, I am okay and, as I said, working everyday."

* * *

Author's Observations:

Perhaps the most obvious and important observation that I was able to make was the attitude of hope and confidence on the part of the patients who were there for treatment. They had no doubt about being cured or at least improving to a point where they could live normally again. This contrasted with what I had observed back home during my wife's short illness.

The pain, despair, lack of hope, nausea, loss of hair and almost total confinement to home, mostly in bed or on a couch, were in sharp contrast to the atmosphere which existed at American Biologics Hospital.

Patients were joyful, enthusiastic, laughing, smiling to a point where one had to remember that this was a clinic to treat people who had been judged terminally ill.

As the word spread that I was interviewing patients, several came to me asking that I interview them also. Because of a schedule to visit several other clinics in the San Diego, Tijuana area, there just was not enough time to talk with all who wanted to tell their story.

On one of the trips to the clinic, a lady sat next to me who was going for treatment. She also had been told in her home location that the medical establishment could do no more in her case. She was not in good spirits, nor did she reflect the hope and confidence I had seen in most other patients. She was aware how many of the clinic patients had been given back a quality of life, and said, "They are the lucky ones."

I would have liked to have followed the results of her treatment. She declined to give me her name so I am unable to know the final outcome. But I now believe that the patient's attitude has a lot to do with whether or not a cure is achieved, or at least, an ability to maintain some quality of life. With this in mind, I do not have a great deal of hope that her treatment was successful.

While I was a skeptic at first, I am convinced that negative thoughts can be a major deterrent to well being. I wonder if some doctors realize how their attitude toward patients can negate any possibility of healing, no matter what the treatment.

Anyone who visits this clinic, although it has the capabilities of many modern hospitals, would hardly know that it is a place of medical treatment and healing. Watching everyone in the dining room, I was aware that conversations were constant, people were animated and laughing, and everyone apparently had a hearty appetite. I could see no discouraging evidence in either the atmosphere or the people to indicate these patients had been told that modern medicine could do no more for them and they were going to die.

The prospect of hope for life, the consequent joy of the patients and their loved ones stimulated an atmosphere of happiness that was absolutely amazing to me. Perhaps this in combination with the treatment, the absence of nausea, the reduction of pain - much of which results from chemotherapy and radiation - all combine to help the body fight the disease. I also think it is most important that the treatment addresses a need to eliminate negative thoughts.

American Biologics Hospital maintains a list of patients who have been successfully treated and who are willing to answer questions. Detailed information is available from the hospital. The contact point for the Alivizatos Treatment at The American Biologics Hospital is Kathleen Jewett. The office is in San Ysidro, California, and the phone numbers are as follows:

Kathleen Jewett (San Ysidro)   1-800-262-0212
Her home number is -   1-800-676-4714
The American Biologics Hospital, call Juan at:
1-800-785-0490 (USA) or 011-526-681-3171 (Mexico)

* * *

OASIS HOSPITAL
TIJUANA, MEXICO

The Oasis Hospital was founded by Dr. Ernesto Contreras, M.D., who developed an approach which he called Total Care.

It was designed to combat cancer and improve the quality of life. The doctor's philosophy in developing this approach, according to hospital literature, recognized that a whole person has physical, mental and spiritual needs. Thus, the treatment effectively treats the entire patient; body, mind and spirit.

The Contreras Total Care Approach is based on two fundamental principles:

1. First do no harm (Hippocrates) (Part of the oath all medical doctors take)
2. Love your patient as yourself "(Dr. Contreras' medical application of Christ's commandment)"

An appointment was made for me to visit the Oasis Hospital on a Sunday morning. Transportation was via a van in which out-patients were being taken to the hospital. I was able to chat with some of the people on the van as the trip took about 30 minutes or more. The attitude of everyone was cheerful and upbeat.

One lady who appeared to be in her 60's had been taken to the hospital on a stretcher. She was diagnosed with lung cancer which had spread to her back and spine. However, she had walked to the van and told me that except for being a little weak, her condition was greatly improved.

The van, provided by the motel where most of the out-patients were staying, stopped at the American Biologics Hospital to drop people off there. It then continued to the Oasis Hospital, located a greater distance from the American border.

I found the trip to be very scenic, plus providing some visions of life in Tijuana. I was surprised when at one point we were so high we could see tall buildings in San Diego.

106

The hospital, a multi-story, modern, glass walled building was not really what I expected to see. It looked more like one of the new, medium-rise buildings in a major United States city.

Inside, everything seemed to be operating very efficiently and everyone was busy, yet courteous and anxious to show off their facility. The chief of staff, with whom I had an interview, was with a patient and would be available within the hour.

I experienced an unprecedented willingness by the entire staff, doctors and nurses who handled the medical procedures, to spend time and patiently explain what they were doing. Dr. Contreras was ill at the time I was there but after I had returned to my home, I received a very gracious letter from him expressing regret at not being available. He mentioned in the letter he was writing a book on his own life and experiences.

His philosophy is evident in his previously published response to the question of why patients call the Contreras Center, "An Oasis of Hope." "It is probably because patients are not finding promising solutions in the world of conventional medicine. I am not saying that conventional medication does not work, but the application of the medicine is critical. If the patient is ignored, and the focus of the therapy is the disease, the quality of life can easily be destroyed. We focus on the patient. People that find hope with us have experienced a therapy that is uplifting not only to the immune system abut also to the spirit."

Since 1963, more than 40,000 Americans have sought the care of Doctor Contreras. While the Oasis Hospital provides a variety of physical treatments, there is just as much emphasis on building up the mind and the spirit. All three are required to combat effectively any disease that has invaded the body. He believes any negative thoughts or suggestions, from within or the outside, have a negative effect on the ability of treatment to build up the body's natural defenses.

I was escorted throughout the hospital, top to bottom, with a great deal of pride shown by hospital personnel during the tour. A pharmacy, located in the lowest level, was well stocked and managed by a licensed attendant.

The hospital featured attractively-decorated rooms for in-patients as well as every kind of up- to-date equipment one would expect to find in a modern hospital. It offered the availability of surgical procedures, tests, chemotherapy and radiation.

The facility is run by doctors, all licensed and graduates of legitimate medical colleges. Nurses also are registered graduates. Pride in the facility was obvious and impressive. The staff expressed both pride in what they were doing and interest in patients as human beings, not as clinical statistics.

During the tour, we were given information on the clinic as well as a video explaining the concept of the clinic. It was founded by Dr. Ernesto Contreras, Sr., M.D., in 1963 to provide alternative as well as conventional (if necessary) treatment for cancer patients.

Included in a packet I was given on the center was information about cancer in the United States. A brochure stated it is estimated that:

- 1.3 million new cases of cancer would occur in 1996.
- 600,000 would die in the same year.
- Since President Nixon and the NCI declared war on cancer in 1972, more than 29 billion dollars has been spent and more than 10 million Americans have died of the disease.

After the tour, which included patient-treatment areas, I was escorted to the office of the chief of staff, Dr. Antonio Jimenez Tapia, M.D. The young doctor was in no hurry and discussed in detail the treatments available, times and schedules. One of the important factors that he stressed was the amount of time the doctors gave patients on a scheduled basis. This partly was because of concern for the mental and spiritual well being of the patient, as well as medical treatment.

The hospital does not reject the philosophy of conventional medicine in combination with its standard treatments, and for that reason has both the willingness and capabilities to provide it.

At the conclusion of the interview with the chief of staff, Dr. Tapia, he said if I had any questions at all, while there or after leaving, I should contact him. There was never any hurry on his part, even though I know he had duties to perform and patients to see.

It was a beautiful, warm morning in Tijuana and patients were outside enjoying the sunshine. Many were on IV's but were able to take their packets of medication and stands with them so they could continue to receive treatment intravenously. I did not detect any feelings of doom or despair in the attitudes of patients being treated. The scene provided insight into how the desperately ill can look at life with hope and anticipation. I could not help but consider it a tragedy that people angrily and loudly reject such places without first investigating them as I was doing.

The van arrived to go back to the motel and provided another scenic ride. By the time we reached the International Motor Inn located in San Ysidro, California, it was already mid-afternoon. The day had been spent in a most interesting and pleasant environment.

As I reflected on past events and the new information I was learning, several thoughts crossed my mind. Modern science and medicine have progressed in many ways over the years. Technology has moved ahead at a fantastic pace. New equipment and procedures are evolving so swiftly it seems obsolescence occurs by nightfall to that which became available in the morning.

Yet, it seems little thought is given to building mental and spiritual outlooks. Without this, there is little opportunity for a person to feel the most important ingredient in healing, and that is hope. Do we progress but lose sight of the human factor? It seems that way?

At the Oasis Hospital I experienced that philosophy of Total Care. Practiced in a most serious way. It recognizes the human factor and all the needs of the body to be able to mount its own defenses. Treatment of the person, indeed, must recognize that it consists of medical, mental and spiritual factors. All are of equal importance if the body is to fight its own battle against disease.

The Oasis Hospital maintains a list of patients who are willing to discuss their treatment. This information may be obtained directly from Oasis Hospital. For information on the treatments that are available, the phone number is toll free:

1-800-700-1850

* * *

LIVINGSTON FOUNDATION MEDICAL CENTER
SAN DIEGO, CALIFORNIA

The Livingston Foundation Medical Center was founded in 1969 by the late Dr. Virginia C. Livingston in the Loma Portal area of San Diego. According to literature provided by the Center, Dr. Livingston was an internationally recognized clinician, healer and prominent medical researcher who devoted her entire life to the study of the body's immune system and its relationship to a variety of human diseases.

Much of her findings have been published. Some of her books which I have read include: Cancer - A New Breakthrough, The Conquest of Cancer, and The Microbiology of Cancer.

In general, the medical profession seems to have agreed with some of her research and conclusions but have also violently not agreed with other aspects.

She states on page four in her book, "Cancer: A New Breakthrough", that she believes the causative agent is the hidden killer - Cryptocides. In her book, "The Conquest of Cancer," she stated, "The microbe I discovered to be acid-fast and classified as Progenitor Cryptocides is a bacillus that is a first cousin to the bacilli that cause tuberculosis and leprosy."

She also stated, "This microbe is present in all of our cells, and it is only our immune systems that keep it suppressed."

On page five, she says further that the purpose of the book is to relate the disease of cancer to an infectious agent, Progenitor Cryptocides, and to describe how this hidden or occult infection produces the many forms of the disease.

She believed that it was incontrovertible that the cancer disease results in the loss of immunity, yet it is treated with radiation and drugs which destroy immunity. However, she was able to establish her clinic and provide her approach to alternative treatment.

Dr. Livingston's original basis of treatment was to initially culture a urine specimen which was used to prepare an autogenous vaccine. The patient is put on a special nutritional diet. These two approaches in combination were described as being effective against many types of cancer and were the kinds of treatment provided by the Center.

After interviews had been completed at other clinics and hospitals in the San Diego area, I called Livingston Foundation Medical Center. Those with whom I conversed were very cordial and receptive to my visiting the facility. I was able to make an appointment for the following morning.

The facility, as I've already mentioned, is located in the Loma Portal area of San Diego. Since I was not familiar with that area, I was given detailed instructions on how to get to the Center. Instructions on how to find the location were given to me over the telephone to include the approximate amount of time it would take to get there. Travel time was almost exactly as was estimated.

Because the instructions I had been given were so detailed and exact, finding the Center was relatively easy. Arrival was just a few minutes before the scheduled time of the appointment. Center personnel provided a warm and positive greeting.

My visit was to include discussions, a tour of the facility and answers to many questions. All were accomplished in a most professional way by Ms. Linda Parker, the Assistant Director. She was extremely cooperative and was very anxious to provide whatever information was requested. She personally showed me the entire facility. At no time did I feel that there was any rush, or that there was any attempt to hide anything.

The pride in the clinic which was shared by all employees with whom I either chatted or came in contact, was consistent throughout the visit and with all who participated in providing of information and answering questions.

This facility, unlike the ones visited in Tijuana, was more limited in its capacity for patients. The treatment was somewhat different or so it seemed based upon the detailed explanations which were given. Also, in reading Dr. Livingston's books, as I had stated before, I had learned that her beliefs about the cause and nature of cancer led her to adopt an immunological approach to the treatment of cancer. Her immunological treatment programs were based upon models developed during her more than 50 years of research.

However, the belief that it was absolutely essential that a special nutritional diet be utilized was consistent with practically every provider of alternative treatment.

In response to the question as to the numbers who have been treated, it was stated that thousands of patients from around the world have been successfully treated. Dr. Livingston came to believe that any treatment should work with and strengthen the body's own immune system. Some of the immunological enhancement therapies and techniques which were developed by Dr. Livingston include vaccines, diet and nutrition vitamins, psychological counseling, detoxification, use of antibiotics to overcome underlying infections, and traditional drug therapy. Whatever is used must serve as a part of enhancing the immune system.

The success rate was impressive and once more, and this has become my most important conclusion, the stress was that the quality of life was maintained at a much higher level than that provided by conventional methods.

This clinic, like so many medical facilities as well as those M.D.'s who attempt to practice alternative medicine, faces constant harassment. It seems that there is a concerted dedication to destroy anything or anyone not following procedures which are prescribed as accepted, normal treatment by the medical profession.

While no patients were observed or interviewed, the attitude of the staff was one of confidence and pride. This seems typical of every instance of contact with any facility providing alternative treatment. I'm sure that the constant concern of attack and threat by the medical profession must produce a condition of stress for everyone. However, they seem to bear up well, even under such conditions, and that is to their credit.

Ms. Parker told me that hundreds of patients are treated each year. However, the treatment is only available to ambulatory patients. The Center is not equipped to handle patients who require bed care.

In her books, Dr. Livingston had stated that she hoped to raise funds in order to provide on site facilities in which patients could be provided complete treatment including lodging. This worthy effort
did not reach fruition and the Center continues to operate on an out-patient basis.

As was the case with other facilities visited, Livingston Foundation Medical Center was well kept, clean and well lighted. Dr. Livingston's books as well as other reading material are kept in inventory for those who would like to purchase copies.

Ms. Parker mentioned a cook book was being completed for future publication, but a title was not yet finalized. Its recipes will be based on foods which conform to the nutritional needs of human bodies. These needs are primarily for the protection and enhancement of the immune system as well as the maintenance of a healthy body. (See note 1 at the end of this chapter)

There was no attempt to limit my visit. I left only after all my questions had been answered. In particular, but this applies to everyone else at the Center, Ms. Parker actually stimulated questions on my part. My departure was with a feeling of leaving new found friends who were deeply concerned with the welfare of their patients. Here was yet another facility which stressed the body's own defense mechanism. Also, my belief was reinforced that the use of an immunological approach certainly did not destroy the quality of life.

Ms. Parker assured me that if I had any further questions, that I should contact her whenever I felt the need. Since that time, I have had several occasions to correspond with Ms. Parker. Her replies have been prompt and her responses left no doubt that she welcomed my letters.

Information on Livingston Foundation Medical Center and the specialized immune enhancement treatment programs they provide can be obtained by contacting the Medical Center at their toll free number:

1-888-777-7321   or
Internet address: www.livingstonmedcentr.com
E-mail address: lfmc@worldnet.att.net

Comment: For both the Internet and E-mail addresses, all letters should be typed in lower case and there are no spaces.

Note - At the time of this printing, Livingston Foundation has published this book and it is entitled "The Cookbook" by Ana Maria Canales.

* * *

CHAPTER SIXTEEN

Smoking and Addiction

Efforts over the years to convince my wife Meryl to quit smoking were futile. She began with cigarettes when she was in college, and the habit or addiction was continuous for perhaps 50 years, or more.

We all believe, perhaps wishfully, that an important factor in lengthening her life was the fact she stopped smoking once we arrived in Juarez, Mexico, to begin her initial non conventional treatment. I am not aware she smoked a single cigarette while in Juarez.

I believe some of her confidence that she would get well was restored when she started to feel better after the reactions from radiation on her spine and the first round of chemotherapy.

With that restoration of confidence and feeling improved, she apparently was unable to resist the urge to smoke again. Her addiction to smoking was so great that she began going to the bathroom a few times a day in order to light up a cigarette in secret.

Meryl thought she was hiding this from us by burning incense in the bathroom and by constantly spraying a disinfectant. While we had removed all the cigarettes we knew were in the house, she managed to hide perhaps two or more cartons which she smoked over several months.

A day arrived when she probably felt better than at any time since the original diagnosis and any subsequent time. She announced she wanted to try driving around the neighborhood and wanted to do it by herself.

When I questioned what she would do if something happened, she informed me that she would just turn into the curb and stop. I did not have the heart to deny her what she wanted.

I helped her to the car, overjoyed that she seemed so happy to be able to get behind the wheel and drive again. She left waving and had a heart- warming smile on her face.

It occurred to me only after she left that her purpose probably was to purchase cigarettes without my knowing. She had taken a large cloth bag and her purse, insisting the bag made it easy to carry the purse that contained her driver's license.

When she returned about 25 minutes later, I believe her concern about cancer was for the moment, just a dim memory. As I helped her out of the car and into the house, I was looking at her bag quite closely and observed the cloth was filled now where it had sagged when she left.

She wanted to go directly to the bathroom and I knew it was in order to hide what she had purchased. How she managed to get to a store to make the purchase was the question a friend asked later. It would have been impossible for her to get from the car into a store. Her only recourse had to be a drive-through type facility. Obviously, she would not have had to leave the car as an attendant would have brought her purchase to her.

We are all convinced now that Meryl's need for cigarettes was due to the fact that smoking for some people is an all-consuming addiction. It was particularly difficult for me to understand why she was unable to quit. Unrelenting addiction, physically and emotionally, was not a personal problem for me. How could I understand it?

I decided to quit a number of years ago after one of my secretaries complained of my cigarette and cigar smoke. Without another thought and with two boxes of cigars and three cartons of cigarettes in my desk, I stopped and never smoked again. It was not at all a difficult thing for me. Throughout my life, I have never allowed anything other than my mind to take control of my body. Once I had decided, there was little or no desire to start smoking again.

Meryl's efforts, as she had tried to quit several times, were completely ineffective. It is difficult to believe that pain, suffering and knowing that death may be just a matter of time are not enough for some people to overcome the unrelenting desire to continue smoking.

I have found it necessary to understand that we believe what we want to believe.

In her case, and to the very end, she was convinced that smoking was not the cause of her cancer. At the very least, that is what she wanted to believe. The need to smoke was so great that it overcame her common sense and her otherwise extremely strong will.

If the addiction had not had an uncompromising hold on her, the need to continue smoking might not have conquered both her will and her spirit.

Her desire to continue smoking probably made little or no difference in the progress of her cancer. By the time it was diagnosed, it was probably too late to stop.

Perhaps continuing to smoke on a greatly reduced basis may have helped her mental state. Certainly from my knowledge of her previous attempts to quit, the physical pain she always suffered was somewhat concealed by the constant cancer pain.

Although I detest admitting this, I believe her mental outlook and morale improved when she was secretly smoking four to six cigarettes a day, or less. When she was in the hospital, she obviously could not smoke. She was so ill most of her days there, I doubt it was a factor. She was in such great pain and fear that her first thoughts had to be of her condition.

My purpose now in relating Meryl's experience is both to emphasize our belief that tobacco is such an addiction for some people that they continue smoking even when critically ill, and to stress that the tobacco industry should consider taking some responsibility to help find a cancer cure.

* * *

CHAPTER SEVENTEEN

An Idea for the Tobacco Industry

"HELP FIND A CURE FOR LUNG CANCER"

This chapter is set aside for the tobacco industry. It contains an idea which I believe has a great deal of merit in a number of ways. I hope that it receives some serious consideration. If the executives of tobacco companies, tobacco growers and others involved in the many facets of the manufacture of various tobacco products show no interest, I'm sure that many others in our society will.

Shortly after my wife's death, our son, who is an attorney and has never used tobacco products until he started smoking an occasional cigar in recent years, said if his mother had used only one brand of cigarettes during her life, he would have been tempted to join the growing group of suits being filed. His comment triggered my thoughts and several aspects came to mind.

First, he was convinced that cigarettes were the primary cause of lung cancer. Second, he was equally convinced that smoking must be stopped because of his belief that it causes cancer. Now, seeing what his mother had to endure, he has absolutely no tolerance for smoking.

Today, we find that the hazards of smoking have been expanded to include so called second-hand smoke. Throughout the United States, those who do not smoke do not want to be exposed to the smoke of those who do. Smokers are not happy with going outside in sub-freezing weather in order to have a cigarette. I have talked with many people who feel it is unfair to keep attacking the industry. More importantly, and as in the case of my wife, many really do not believe or want to believe, that lung cancer is caused by cigarettes.

However, I think the predominance of thought is that cigarettes are a major cause of lung cancer. That belief dominates the media, government, ex-smokers as well as those who have never smoked. For myself, I think cigarettes trigger lung cancer but it can remain in a dormant stage until some trauma and highly stressful situation occurs which compromises one's immune system. Once the body becomes vulnerable, the cancer is able to become active and there is little or no resistance to its spread.

I am convinced of this for two reasons. One is that many doctors and scientists have written that we all have cancer cells in our bodies which remain inactive until something occurs which triggers them. That happens at a time when the immune system is drastically lowered and the body is no longer able to combat the cancer cells. Once this illness occurs, my belief is that in any illness, including small cell lung cancer, the body's immune system must be restored to its peak condition in order to combat the disease effectively.

At this point, my personal evaluation has brought me to a series of observations, questions and conclusions. I will enumerate them as carefully and as succinctly as possible:

• If in reality, stress is what triggers cancer into becoming active, that should be a beginning point in stopping cancer before it becomes a danger.

• If cigarettes are a basic cause of cancer but the disease does not take hold until stress occurs with an accompanying loss of immunity, then this could give the medical community another prevention tool.

• Lung cancer claims many who never smoked, lived exemplary lives and did not have significant exposure to secondary smoke. Why did they get cancer?

• The EPA claims that Radon is the second greatest cause of lung cancer. I was a member of a committee of engineers who investigated the claims of the danger of Radon. Except for those who have worked in mines and been in close contact with radium which is the source of the gas, we found no positive proof that would substantiate either the claims or the levels which the Environmental Protection Agency states are acceptable concentrations of the gas.

The cigarette industry is taking more than just the brunt of responsibility for lung cancer. It has a legitimate worry about the increasing number of suits being filed and their reaction is not always coordinated. At least, it seems so from media accounts. Something better

118

is needed other than reaction, defensive responses and fighting the ever increasing number of law suits.

• The fighting of litigation as well as the denials of so many accusations of being responsible does not really smooth the waters.

• A sizable portion of our economy depends upon tobacco to survive. If the industry were suddenly stopped, the effect on the economy would be dramatic. However, that does not reduce the death rate, nor the pain and suffering caused by cancer. Nor is it an excuse so that in order for the industry to survive, so many should suffer.

What then should occur which might preserve the industry? One must consider that smoking is a world-wide affliction although one person's belief of an affliction is another person's pleasure. The threat of cancer has not deterred millions of people from continuing to smoke.

Considering these factors, I asked myself what I would do if I had a say in the tobacco industry?. I considered both the industry and the public as well as the response of both the governmental regulating agencies and the medical community. In my thoughts, I gave much consideration to what the responsibility should be of the tobacco industry. Finally, I found that tobacco companies were spending millions of dollars in advertising and in combating both the accusations of causing cancer as well as the many suits in progress.

With these thoughts, I became convinced that the total tobacco industry, since much of the public is convinced that it is responsible for lung cancer, should start considering its role in finding a cure for the disease.

This brought me to a personal conclusion. *IF THE TOBACCO INDUSTRY WERE TO DEVOTE SIGNIFICANT EFFORT AND MONEY INTO A RIFLE APPROACH TO FINDING A CURE FOR LUNG CANCER, SUCH A DECISION WOULD FIND GREAT FAVOR WITH THE PUBLIC. BUT OF GREATER IMPORTANCE, JOINING THE BATTLE TO FIND THE CAUSE AND A CURE WOULD GIVE MANKIND A GREAT GIFT, HOPEFULLY, ENDING THE TERRIBLE PAIN AND SUFFERING OF THOSE WHO FIND THEMSELVES WITH LUNG CANCER.*

The ramifications go further. If a cure were to be found and I am convinced now that we have the tools and intelligence to do so, then the tobacco industry could continue to be a vital part of our economy. The down side is that it would cause some hardship on the medical community.

Portions of hospitals and clinics might be forced into closing. The National Cancer Institute as well as the American Cancer Society could be left with little to do.

THE BOON TO MANKIND OVERCOMES ALL OTHER CONSIDERATIONS.

Although it might sound a little self-centered, I can think of no other action that would receive a more favorable public reaction. This would be great public relations and the greatest of contributions to the health of the people worldwide.

Yet, I would add a word of caution. There are probably many who would view an undertaking of this sort with suspicion. I am sure some people would believe the effort would not be a true adventure into the finding of a cure. Some would want to believe the tobacco industry would use this approach to produce only announcements refuting the role tobacco plays in causing lung cancer. The public has become very suspicious of all that happens in our society. We have good reason to become cynics. After all, how often have we been exposed to an announcement only to discover later that what we thought was factual turned out to be the truth stretched or a plain, downright lie.

The idea then must be publicized in good faith and what is stated must be the absolute truth. Otherwise, it will be just another case of greedy corporations taking advantage of the public.

This comes from a person who stopped smoking many years ago because it distressed others. It comes from one who continues to grieve over the loss of his wife of 44 years, from a person who watched her pain and suffering for the short time she lived, from one who shared her joy in believing the conventional treatment she was receiving would give her more years to enjoy our children and grandsons.

In a world which has seen little progress in finding a cure for lung cancer, and in which the conventional treatment can be worse than the disease, new ideas are needed. How the medical community can hold up its head knowing that surgery, radiation and chemotherapy will only destroy the quality of life for those with small cell lung cancer is beyond me.

Something else is needed where nothing so far has worked. It's time to seek new solutions.

Human nature is beyond the control of our peers, government and legislation. Nothing short of real fear has caused people to avoid harmful practices, and then only some people. Certainly, the obvious failure of prohibition proved that legislation will not stop people from drinking alcoholic beverages. Such attempts to regulate human nature have failed throughout the history of mankind.

It's time for a real effort at a solution. Otherwise, I see no hope in the immediate future for those who will and are facing certain, horrible death.

If anyone is listening, let's stop fighting each other and stop the cause of the fight.

I believe the tobacco industry can become one of the greatest contributors in history to the health of the people of the world. I am optimistic the industry can do what the medical community has as yet been unable to do.

* * *

CHAPTER EIGHTEEN

The Need for Home-Care Education

Stress of Caring for a Terminal Cancer Patient

Once the commitment is made to become the caretaker for the patient at home, it requires a period of time to understand how much is involved. Doctors only tell you about medication and a limited number of general medical responsibilities.

Even after months of taking care of my wife, I was still learning at the time of her death. It amazed me how much doctors took for granted and how much they expected from people who had never faced such awesome responsibility. I learned very quickly to ask one question after another, and to make lists of things I would need to know.

One disturbing problem is the fact that it is not always apparent which questions to ask. Initially I found there were always unanswered questions. I had no idea how great the total scope of home care would be.

Anyone facing a situation similar to ours perhaps can benefit from some of the information our family learned. It may prevent part of the heartbreak and frustration we experienced.

In Mexico, we were given a schedule of the drugs to be taken. They were furnished each day, packaged and marked as to when and under what circumstances they were to be taken.

After our return to Ohio, and as we became more and more involved in radiation and chemotherapy, the drug list began to grow. It reached a point where drugs had to be given at least seven times a day. Rather than trying to memorize this schedule, and because at times my family relieved me while I accomplished other routine tasks, I formulated a drug schedule in my word processor. It had to be modified eight times before it was too late to be needed.

Each modification involved a different format to make it easier for others to follow. After my wife's first stay in the hospital, I became aware I needed to know not only when the drugs should be given, but be able to inform hospital attendants about the drug names and prescriptions.

I have included most of the schedules that my wife had to follow as part of this chapter.

While the patient must endure the physical suffering, the caretaker becomes more and more stressed with the passage of time. The symptoms increase as the patient fails to improve, or if there are setbacks when improved health is expected.

As an example, during my wife's illness, my blood pressure began to increase and fluctuate. I could almost tell what it was going to be, depending upon what was happening with her condition.

Adding to the stress of tending and medicating the patient, is the knowledge that time must be made available to pick up prescriptions, shop for supplies and groceries, and prepare meals (I became a pretty good short order cook) that the patient will find tasteful and nutritional.

In addition, the routine chores we must resolve everyday require time, such as paying bills and handling home maintenance problems. All the multitude of tasks that had to be accomplished daily prior to the illness have to be added to the new priority list of patient care.

We had high winds during my wife's illness which made demands on my time. Huge trees were uprooted, large limbs were ripped off the trees. Also, a roof had to be replaced over the garage, and we needed to install more air conditioning in order to keep my wife comfortable. They became new challenges which added to all the routine requirements of taking care of my wife.

The daily record which I kept and have made part of this book contains a great deal of information which is aside from the care my wife needed. It is included to illustrate just how much occurs, especially when the patient requires twenty-four-hour care.

No two care givers will have the same problems, or should we call them opportunities. In my case, I canceled speeches, radio and television appearances. I suspended all of my consulting work and focused almost completely on my wife, her needs, and keeping the household going.

Many new procedures, devices and descriptions were learned, which re-enforced my belief that the best knowledge is what you learn after you think you know it all. An example was a session I had with a pharmacist after our doctor prescribed Neupogen for the first time. I had to learn how to perform the injections, what precautions to take, verify the proper needles and absorb other bits of information in order to have a degree of confidence in the ability to do properly what needed to be done.

At the conclusion of this book are some sample laboratory blood reports which show the large variations each time another round of chemotherapy was administered. Included also is a scan made of the actual Metaport which was installed early on in the treatment. It was then removed from her chest just two weeks before her demise.

I had no previous experience with blood reports and had to learn what each term meant. Reports list lab results and normal ranges, stating if they are high or low. But the reports lack information for the layman which explain what each item is and what can be is affected.

The red blood counts, as well as the white blood counts, really do not require any special knowledge to understand. But most of the other verbiage was foreign to me. I had little or no idea what was significant and what was not, yet I felt it necessary for me to be aware of all aspects of my wife's varying condition.

I asked for an explanation of some reports from the first nurse who came to the house to take blood. Her answer was that she had forgotten - she was out of nursing school only a few weeks - but said she would bring a book on her next visit which would tell me what I wanted to know. For some reason, she never seemed to remember to bring it. In her defense, my wife told me the nurse had a great ability to insert needles in her arm almost without pain. The book became secondary to that kind of talent.

Looking back now on all that transpired, I am amazed at how much knowledge was required and how I was able to grasp what I had to learn as quickly as I did. If necessity is the mother of invention, then my brain must have invented some new learning paths.

If this information helps reduce the panic and distress for others, the effort to assemble and write this will be worthwhile. One very serious conclusion at which I have arrived has to do with those who deal in medicine on an everyday basis. Someone ought to put together in simple form, the basic things for which the caretaker must take responsibility. I hope that this book is a start.

* * *

MEDICATION AS OF APRIL 18, 1996

TYPE - FOR PAIN
   ORAMORPHONE, 15 MG - SMALL WHITE TABLET
       1 PILL IN MORNING WHENEVER SHE GETS UP
       2 PILLS AT NIGHT WHEN SHE GOES TO BED

PAIN BREAKTHROUGH (ROXANOL - 20MG)
       IN CASE OF PAIN DURING TIME BETWEEN ORAMORPHONE,
       GIVE 1/2 DROPPER IN JUICE EVERY 2 HOURS
  (IMPORTANT) TO PREVENT UPSET STOMACH, TAKE WITH FOOD OR MILK)

TYPE - FOR NAUSEA
   METOCLOPRAMIDE, 10 MG - SMALL WHITE TABLET
   (THIS IS THE SAME AS REGLAN)
       1 TABLET BEFORE MEALS
       1 TABLET AT BEDTIME

NOTE - MEDICATION CONSTANTLY CHANGES SO THERE ARE MANY BOTTLES WITH
TABLETS AND CAPSULES WHICH I HAVE PUT IN A WHITE BAG. THESE ARE ITEMS WHICH   HAVE BEEN PRESCRIBED PREVIOUSLY AND NOT USED NOW. THE CURRENT PRESCRIBED MEDICATION IS AS SHOWN ABOVE.   AS THIS CHANGES, THESE INSTRUCTIONS WILL BE CHANGED ACCORDINGLY.

Original   SUPPLEMENTS

TYPE	AM	NOON	PM
VITAMIN A-E EMULSION	X	X	X
(5 DROPS IN JUICE - STIR WELL)			
(USE VERY LITTLE JUICE)			
CAT'S SLAW - UNA DE GATO	X	X	X
(2 EA 1/2 HOUR BEFORE MEALS)			
(THE ITEMS MARKED * ARE PACKAGED			
TOGETHER IN ZIP BAGS)			
*ENZYME T (2 CAPSULES-3 TIMES DAILY)	X	X	X
*UNA DE GATO (2 CAPS-3 TIMES DAILY)	X	X	X
(30 min before meals)			
*THYMUS PMG (1 TABLET-3 TIMES DAILY)	X	X	X
*AMIGDALN (1 TABLET-2 TIMES DAILY)	X		X
*COENZYME Q10 (1 CAP-3 TIMES DAILY)	X	X	X

TYPE	AM	NOON	PM
*ECHINACEA (1 CAP-3 TIMES DAILY)	X	X	X
(THE ABOVE ARE PACKAGED IN ZIP BAGS			
AND MARKED AM, NOON AND PM)			
SHARK CARTILAGE (3 CAPS 3 TIMES DAILY) X		X	X
(30 MINUTES AFTER MEALS)			

SCHEDULE 4   CURRENT MEDICATION AS OF MAY 8, 1996

TYPE - FOR PAIN
         ORAMORPHONE, 15 MG - SMALL WHITE TABLET
            1 PILL AT NIGHT WHEN SHE GOES TO BED
         ROXICET
            1 TABLET EVERY 6 HOURS AS NEEDED
            CAN GIVE MORE IF NEEDED
TYPE - FOR NAUSEA
         USE COMPAZINE, UP TO 4 OR 5 DAILY IF NEEDED
         (GREENISH TABLETS)
         IF NAUSEA IS SEVERE, USE ZOFRAIN, 1 EVERY 8 HOURS
TYPE - FOR APPETITE
         MARINOL - 2 TABLETS DAILY
            1 BEFORE LUNCH AND 1 BEFORE SUPPER
TYPE - CHEMOTHERAPY
         VEPESID - 3 CAPSULES DAILY AFTER LUNCH, THURS, FRI, SAT, &
         SUN
            MAY 9, 10, 11, 12 (MUST KEEP REFRIGERATED)
TYPE - SHOTS
         NEUPOGEN - 1 INJECTION DAILY ABOUT 1 PM STARTING
         TUESDAY, MAY 14 FOR 10 DAYS (MUST KEEP
         REFRIGERATED)

NOTE - WILL NUMBER EACH NEW SET OF INSTRUCTIONS. THIS ONE IS NUMBER 4. THE NEXT ONE WILL BE NUMBER 5. EACH NEW SCHEDULE SUPERSEDES ALL PREVIOUS SCHEDULES. BE SURE TO CHECK BOTH SCHEDULE NUMBER AND DATE SO THAT YOU ARE WORKING ON CURRENT PRESCRIPTION SCHEDULE.

NOTE 2 - NURSE IS CURRENTLY COMING ON MONDAY AND THURSDAY TO DRAW BLOOD, CHECK BLOOD PRESSURE, PULSE AND TEMPERATURE. BLOOD RESULTS CAN BE PICKED UP AT 181 GRANVILLE STREET, NEXT TO FIFITH-THIRD BANK. CLINIC IS LOCATED IN BASEMENT, FIRST DOOR ON RIGHT. ALL BLOOD TEST RESULTS CAN BE PICKED UP AT 181 GRANVILLE STREET, NEXT TO FIFTH-THIRD BANK. CLINIC IS LOCATED IN THE BASEMENT, FIRST DOOR ON RIGHT. ALL BLOOD TEST RESULTS ARE IN A FOLDER WITH THE LATEST ON TOP.

* * *

SCHEDULE_5   CURRENT MEDICATION AS OF JUNE 14, 1996

DRUG	BREAKFAST	LUNCH	DINNER	BEDTIME
COLACE (LAXATIVE)	X		X	
ZOFRAN (NAUSEA)	X	X	X	
ZOLOFT (DEPRESSION)	X			
MEGACE (APPETITE)	X X	X X	X X	X X
METOCLOPRAMIDE (REGLAN) (30_MIN_BEFORE_EATING)	X	X	X	X
PRILOSEC (30 MIN BEFORE EATING BREAKFAST) (BEDTIME_IS_OK)	X			X

DELTASONE   (NO LONGER USED)

	BREAKFAST	LUNCH	DINNER	BEDTIME
ORAMORPH (ACTUAL PRESCRIPTION IS 1 AT WAKEUP AND 1 AT BEDTIME) (SHE HAS BEEN TAKING ONLY 1 AT_BEDTIME)				X

EMLA   (SALVE) - A LITTLE ON METAPORT 30 TO 45 MINUTES BEFORE NURSE COMES   TO TAKE BLOOD)

*START ON JUNE,15

NEUPOGEN_(BY_INJECTION_ONCE_A_DAY_AFTER_CHEMOTHERAPY)____
*_(10_TOTAL)

EPOGEN_(BY_INJECTION_MON-WEDS-FRI-_START_6-17-96)

ROXANOL (LIQUID PAIN RELEASE. MAY BE TAKEN EVERY 3-4 HOURS AS NEEDED   FOR BREAKTHROUGH PAIN) (THIS HAS NOT BEEN USED SINCE 24 MAY WHEN SHE_WAS_RELEASED_FROM_HOSPITAL)

SUPPLEMENTS	BREAKFAST	LUNCH	DINNER
ENZYME T	X	XX	XX
AMYGDALIN	X		X
ECHINACEA	X		X
IRON (400G)	X	* TAKE ONLY IF NEEDED WITH	

A

FULL GLASS OF WATER

	BREAKFAST	LUNCH	DINNER
VIT B COMPLEX	X		
POTASSIUM	X (IF BLOOD RESULTS SHOW IT IS NEEDED)		

CALCIUM-MAG   X (IF BLOOD RESULTS SHOW IT IS NEEDED)

LOW IMMUNITY AFTER CHEMOTHERAPY WILL BE 10-14 DAYS AFTER TREATMENT HAS BEEN GIVEN

SCHEDULE_6   CURRENT_MEDICATION_AS_OF_AUGUST_9,_1996

DRUG	BREAKFAST	LUNCH	DINNER	BEDTIME
COLACE - 100 MG ____(LAXATIVE)	X		X	
ZOFRAN - 8 MG ____(NAUSEA)	X	X	X	
ZOLOFT - 100 MG ____(DEPRESSION)	X			
MEGACE - 40 MG ____(APPETITE)	X X	X X	X X	X X
METOCLOPRAMIDE (REGLAN)	X	X	X	X
(30_MIN_BEFORE EATING)	X	X	X	
PRILOSEC - 20MG (30 MIN BEFORE EATING BREAKFAST)* (BEDTIME_IS_OK) 15MG TABS	X			X
ORAMORPH -(PAIN) (30 MINUTES BEFORE EATING)	X			X
FERROUS SULFATE 324MG TABS-30 MIN BEFORE BREAKFAST (IRON SUPPLEMENT)	X			

EMLA   (SALVE) A LITTLE ON METAPORT 45 MINUTES OR MORE BEFORE NURSE TAKES_BLOOD)
1 ML VIAL-300MCG
NEUPOGEN_(BY_INJECTION_ONCE_A_DAY_FOR_10_DAYS_AFTER CHEMOTHERAPY)_____1 VIAL - 10,000U/ML
EPOGEN_(BY_INJECTION_MON-WEDS-FRI-_**START_6-17-96)**
ROXANOL (LIQUID PAIN RELEASE. MAY BE TAKEN EVERY 3-4 HOURS AS NEEDED FOR BREAKTHROUGH PAIN)

SUPPLEMENTS -	BREAKFAST	LUNCH	DINNER	BEDTIME

ENZYME T	X	XX	XX
AMYGDALIN	X		X
ECHINACEA	X		X
VIT B COMPLEX	X		
POTASSIUM	X (IF BLOOD RESULTS SHOW IT IS NEEDED)		
CALCIUM-MAG	X (IF BLOOD RESULTS SHOW IT IS NEEDED)		

LOW IMMUNITY AFTER CHEMOTHERAPY WILL BE 10-14 DAYS AFTER START OF EACH ROUND

SCHEDULE_7   CURRENT_MEDICATION_AS_OF_AUGUST_20,_1996

DRUG_____	BREAKFAST	LUNCH	DINNER	BEDTIME
METOCLOPRAMIDE (REGLAN) - 10MG TABS (NAUSEA - STOMACH DISORDERS) 30 MINUTES BEFORE EATING AND/OR AT BEDTIME)				
PRILOSEC - 20MG CAPS (REDUCE STOMACH ACID)	X			
MEGACE - - (200MG OR 5ML)(LIQUID) (APPETITE)(SMALL PLASTIC CUPS)	X	X	X	X
FERROUS SULFATE - 324MG TABS (IRON FOR RED BLOOD)	X	X		
ORAMORPH - 15MG TABS (PAIN) (30 MIN BEFORE BREAKFAST)	X			XX
BACTRIM - TABS, 800-160, (ANTI-BIOTIC) (BREAK TABS IN	X	X		
HALF TO MAKE SWALLOWING EASIER) **(STOP TAKING 8-25)** (TAKE AFTER MEALS)				
COLACE - 100MG CAPS (LAXATIVE)	X	X		
ZOFRAN - 8MG TABS (NAUSEA) (AS NEEDED)	X	X	X	
ZOLOFT - 100MG TABS (DEPRESSION)	X			
LACTULOSE - 30CC LIQUID (LAXATIVE)	X			

SPECIAL INSTRUCTIONS:
ROXANOL (HALF DROPPER IN JUICE)
(PAIN BREAKTHROUGH) (EVERY 3 HOURS IF NEEDED)
NEUPOGEN - 1ML VIAL, 300MCG

(INJECTION-ONCE A DAY FOR 10 DAYS BEGINNING DAY AFTER END OF CHEMO)
EPOGEN_- 10,000/ML VIALS
(INJECTION MON, WEDS, FRI AS NEEDED FROM BLOOD RESULTS)

SUPPLEMENTS: (IF NEEDED)	BREAKFAST	LUNCH	DINNER	BEDTIME
ENZYME T	X	X	X	
AMYGDALIN	X		X	
ECHINACEA	X	X	X	
VIT B COMPLEX	X		X	
POTASSIUM	X			
CALCIUM-MAGNESIUM	X		X	

*******IMPORTANT***** LOW BLOOD LEVELS WILL BE 10-14 DAYS AFTER START OF EACH ROUND OF CHEMOTHERAPY. DURING THIS PERIOD, PATIENT WILL BE SUSCEPTIBLE TO INFECTION. NO FRESH FRUIT OR VEGETABLES AT THIS TIME

SCHEDULE_8   CURRENT_MEDICATION_AS_OF_AUGUST_30,_1996_

DRUG_____ _____	BREAKFAST	LUNCH	DINNER	BEDTIME
METOCLOPRAMIDE (REGLAN) (10MG TABS)(NAUSEA - STOMACH DISORDERS) (30 MIN BEFORE EATING AND/OR BEDTIME)	X	X	X	X
PRILOSEC - 20MG CAPS (REDUCE STOMACH ACID)	X			
MEGACE - 200MG OR 5 ML - LIQUID	X	X	X	X
(APPETITE)(SMALL PLASTIC CUPS)				
FERROUS SULFATE - 324MG TABS (IRON FOR RED BLOOD)		X		
ORAMORPH - 15MG TABS (PAIN)	X			XX
BACTRIM - TABS, 800-160, (ANTI-BIOTIC) (BREAK TABS IN HALF TO MAKE SWALLOWING EASIER)(STOP_8-25)				
AFTER_MEALS:				
COLACE - 100MG CAPS	X			X
(LAXATIVE)				
ZOFRAN - 8MG TABS (NAUSEA) (AS NEEDED	X	X	X	

ZOLOFT - 100MG TABS   X
    (DEPRESSION)
LACTULOSE - 30CC LIQUID   X
      (LAXATIVE) (AS NEEDED)

SPECIAL INSTRUCTIONS:

ROXANOL (HALF DROPPER IN JUICE)
(PAIN BREAKTHROUGH)
(EVERY 3 HOURS IF NEEDED)
NEUPOGEN - 1ML VIAL, 300MCG
(INJECTION-ONCE A DAY FOR 10 DAYS
BEGINNING DAY AFTER END OF CHEMO)
EPOGEN_- 10,000/ML VIALS
(INJECTION MON, WEDS, FRI AS NEEDED FROM BLOOD RESULTS)

SUPPLEMENTS: (IF NEEDED)

ENZYME T	X	X	X
AMYGDALIN	X	X	
ECHINACEA	X	X	X
VIT B COMPLEX	X		X
POTASSIUM	X		
CALCIUM-MAGESIUM	X	X	

*****IMPORTANT***** LOW BLOOD LEVELS WILL BE 10-14 DAYS AFTER START OF EACH ROUND OF CHEMOTHERAPY. DURING THIS PERIOD, PATIENT WILL BE SUSCEPTIBLE TO INFECTION. NO FRESH FRUIT OR VEGETABLES AT THIS TIME

* * *

CHAPTER NINETEEN

If I Could To It Do Over Again

Looking back with the wisdom of hindsight, I now have the belief and regret of knowing that I would have done a number of things differently. But that is easily said, having gone through this terrible experience of shock and grief at the beginning. Then came a succession of hope, grief, fear, disappointment, dismay, hope again, stress and finally, the end.

Before I proceed further, it must be understood that any decision was not mine alone. My wife certainly had to agree and have hope in whatever we decided.

I believe now that the time spent in Mexico was beneficial in that it does not appear from x-rays that the lung tumor grew during the time we were there. We are not sure how effective the treatment might have been, as her condition at the time was so painful that a great deal of the normal treatment was not administered. However, we were both firmly convinced that her total system, especially kidneys and liver, were brought to excellent condition. Upon our return and after tests were made, we were told by all the doctors involved with her treatment that her kidneys and liver were healthy and in excellent condition.

The pain my wife was experiencing in her legs was a great deterrent to any effective treatment. Finally, surgery was prescribed in Mexico to remove the lesion from her spine that was causing the pain in her legs. After consultation with other doctors, and our son and daughter, we decided to return home and attempt to destroy the lesion with radiation.

From my experience resulting from Meryl's cancer and the resulting gut feelings, I now believe that it would have been better to attack the lesion prior to attempting alternative treatment. This is because initially the pain was bearable and not debilitating. Also, I think that it would have been better to accept only two rounds of chemotherapy. At the same time, trying some of the alternative remedies, as well as concentrating on building up the immune system, might have aided the conventional treatment in combating the cancer. Since her oncologist would not grant me an interview, his opinion is therefore not available. In his words, he stated that he would not be part of an expose and until he had read the book, he would not grant an interview.

A very distressful conclusion at which I have arrived is the dichotomy of trying to battle cancer with a method which also destroys the immune system. What seems obvious to me as a layman doesn't seem to enter into conventional medical thinking. If indeed, the immune system is the most important factor in combating all kinds of disease, how can we accept a program which works against the ability of the body to defend itself. Such is the case with conventional treatment.

It was only after the first rounds of radiation and chemotherapy that I realized with dismay that conventional treatment causes a drastic reduction in the immune system. After each treatment of chemotherapy and during radiation, the immune system is depressed to a point where the greatest concern is infection. Yet, nothing is prescribed to help maintain the immune system other than injections of Neupogen to help build up the white cells and the associated chemistry.

In other words, the use of radiation and chemotherapy destroys for a time the ability of the body to fight cancer. That doesn't make sense because it is gone when it is need most.

From discussions, experience and resulting conclusions, my feeling of what to do as long as conventional treatment is being administered would be to supplement with all known procedures to keep the immune system as high as possible. Thus, I would consider as many of the published treatments as possible. These would include shark cartilage, flaxseed oil, microbiotics, laetrile, etc. At the same time, I would check the levels of calcium, magnesium, sodium, iron, etc., and supplement as needed. From our experience with her battle against cancer, the only time I felt that some attention was paid to levels of minerals, etc., was when she was hospitalized. And perhaps the most important consideration of all is to establish a nutritional diet as prescribed by MD's such as Drs. Binzel and Pinkham.

During this time, I would contact as many of the M.D.'s and clinics as possible who provide alternative treatment. Depending upon what the conditions might be after two rounds of chemotherapy, I would decide on the next course of action. The one thing I would not do, especially if the disease is small cell lung cancer which has metastisized or spread, would be to continue conventional treatment. Again, this is my personal opinion resulting from experience and interviews.

I wish now that we had done these things. But she developed great faith in the oncologist who was treating her. This caused a fear in me that if I did anything to disrupt the course of her treatment, she would get worse or die. I did nothing to cause any change in the type of treatment she was getting. In the meantime, I carried out all the responsibilities needed for home care, such as checking her blood results, providing her with whatever supplements were below normal and the constant taking of pulse, temperature and blood pressure.

In the case of some of the alternative treatment that was available, we learned the identity of one gentleman who had gone to a clinic in Tijuana, Mexico. He had made this decision after experiencing a number of rounds of chemotherapy. My son was able to reach and talk with him personally. This man is now leading a normal life. My son asked him about the treatment. His response to the question was, "I can only judge by results". "Since the treatment there, I am working everyday, feel fine and there is no sign of lung cancer."

For those of us who are not medically trained and educated, we have no other system of measurement other than results.

I must repeat again my utter disbelief and dismay at the entire concept of radiation and chemotherapy. While it is understood that the object of this treatment is to kill cancer cells, they are both poisons to the body and they also kill good cells. Worse, as stated previously, they cause the immune system to drop to a point where the body is an open invitation to infection. In this condition, the immune system is unable to attack the cancer cells. This aspect of treatment is certainly not understood and is beyond comprehension to me.

Finally, during the weeks of my wife's illness, I found that some medical people had never heard of certain items of non-conventional treatment that were available. While I won't go into this in detail, this did leave me with two thoughts. One, none of this seems to be taught in medical school. Second, after entering into practice, doctors apparently are too busy to investigate non-conventional considerations.

Let me make sure that my points to consider are clear. Now that I know what will normally happen in the case of this disease, the apprehension that the cancer will worsen or cause death is no longer a factor. The certainty of death now becomes a comfort in deciding what to do.

To put it another way, had we opted for alternative treatment after the second round of chemotherapy and she had died, I now know that she would have died anyway. So the terrible guilt that would have existed, knowing what I know now, is gone. But before the fact, we had no way of knowing this. *However, the medical world does know this and could approach the total treatment differently.*

If those in the medical profession read this book and take exception to what has been said, I would not be surprised. But then, I would respond by saying: How can one in good conscience - knowing the pain that will be inflicted upon the patient, knowing death is almost certain in a very short time, knowing the huge cost of a an extra few days or weeks of life and knowing the fairly certain path the disease will take - allow such procedures which seem to be inhumane and without hope?

* * *

CHAPTER TWENTY

Books, References and Other Publications

The list of various references that have been published is quite lengthy. Whether or not they contain information that would address the subject of small cell lung cancer can only be determined by reviewing them all. Such a task is probably a virtual impossibility.

Therefore, I am only listing some publications with which I am familiar. They should provide a beginning for those who find they want to know more than just the information that they receive from normal medical sources.

BOOKS:

Choices in Healing by Michael Lerner
Cancer Therapy by Ralph W. Moss, PhD
Remarkable Recovery by Caryle Hirshberg & Marc Ian Barasch
Cancer Cure by Gary L. Schine with Ellen Berlinsky, PhD
Living with Lung Cancer by Barbara G. Cox, M.A., Ed.S.
David C. Carr, M.D.   Robert E. Lee, M.D.
Questioning Chemotherapy by Ralph W. Moss, PhD
Alive and Well by Philip E. Binzel, Jr., M.D.
Flaxseed (Linseed) Oil and the Power of Omega-3 by
Ingeborg M. Johnston, C.N.   James R. Johnston, PhD
Sharks Don't Get Cancer by Dr. I. William Lane Linda Comac
Sharks Still Don't Get Cancer by Dr. I. William Lane
Prescription for Nutritional Healing by James F. Balch, M.D.
 Phyllis A. Balch, C.N.C.
What Are Clinical Trials All About? U.S. Department of Health and Human Services
Eating Hints for Cancer Patients   National Cancer Institute
Chemotherapy and You   National Cancer Institute

Radiation Therapy and You - National Cancer Institute
What You Should Know About Nutrition for Active Lifestyles
by Dr. Earl Mindell
The Cookbook (Livingston Foundation) - Ana Maria Canales

Publications and References:

A Patient's Guide to the Vena Tech LGM Vena Cava Filter
R. Braun Medical - Vena Tech Division
National Cancer Institute

* * *

CHAPTER TWENTY-ONE

SOME THOUGHTS AND CONCLUSIONS

In my consideration of all the factors during the time I have spent visiting clinics, interviewing doctors, reading everything I could find, listening to documentaries on radio and television, certain opinions have been formed.

I have to ask myself why the world of science and medicine are so defensive and angry when the subject of alternative treatment is raised. The first response which I have heard so many times is, "there is no scientific evidence that this or that treatment works". My reaction is, "what about human evidence". I know now that conventional treatment is a death warrant for a person with metastatic, small cell lung cancer. That person will have just a short time to live but with all quality of life destroyed.

Why is it that the robotic treatment of this type of cancer is continued, knowing that radiation and chemotherapy will destroy all quality of life. If the first part of the Hippocratic Oath is, "I will do no harm", then I believe that the very basis of the practice of medicine is being violated. What will happen is predictable in 95% of patients, yet everything imaginable is done which adds to the suffering and discomfort of the patient. Worse, the treatment destroys the body's ability to fight the disease.

I've observed countless X-rays, bone scans, broncoscopies, MRI's, bodies which are covered with needle marks, accepted procedures which require additional and expensive counter-procedures for them to be effective, etc. The Metaport for example is costly and not dependable to perform as advertised. To a patient already bearing more than a human should, adding to this suffering leaves me extremely frustrated and disappointed.

When I asked the question, "Where is the scientific evidence that proves this treatment is effective", the answer I usually get is that it is the only treatment available to conventional medicine. Yet, this practice is continued knowing that not only is the patient doomed but that a great deal of suffering will be added by the treatment.

It is important to understand that I believe that doctors do what they have been trained to do with the only tools that the medical profession allows them to use. I remember one time when I asked an intern about a certain supplement. He told me that he had never heard of it. His further comment was that they don't teach that in medical school.

Perhaps the strangest revelation in all this is the fact that in every case of alternative treatment, there was always the attitude that if surgery, chemotherapy or radiation were necessary, they should be made available. However, in every case of conversations with those who practiced conventional medicine, I heard nothing but angry ridicule of anything that varied from acceptable standards by the American Medical Profession. This angry defensive attitude has caused me to wonder how those who have taken the Hippocratic Oath seem to be blind to the fact that in some cases, they "do harm" but justify it in a way that escapes my limited logic.

In conclusion, I have one major belief. The best treatment for any disease especially cancer is to bring the body's own immune system to a point where it is the first line of protection. This then leads me to believe that the medical profession must find a line of conventional treatment which enhances rather than destroys the immune system. Chemotherapy and radiation do just the opposite.

* * *

CHAPTER TWENTY-TWO

DANIEL AND MICHELE ABRAHAM

After Michele and Daniel had reviewed the first draft of the book, I sat down with them to discuss any comments they might have on the information included and to hear their own recollections. After a few minutes of discussion, I felt that it might be a good idea to tape the conversation, with the idea of adding their remarks to the book. What follows is a transcript of the their reflections and feelings.

They were both very much concerned and involved with their Mother. I have always felt that there was an unusual closeness in the entire family and especially so between our children and Meryl. Thus, during her terminal illness, their support and involvement were extremely important. How they felt and reacted during this time is very pertinent to the purpose of this book.

Here then is their actual conversation:

MICHELE:

When you have facts, you are able to deal with a life threatening situation better. But when you have confusion about what the facts are, it's a horrible feeling, especially when it's someone you are close to and love dearly. I have to guess that is pretty common.

If someone had all the answers, it probably would be clear and there would be less confusion. So little is known so that I can understand it only to a degree. It's such a business (for the medical profession). They are so overloaded with patients, that I don't believe doctors are in a position to give individual patients the kind of care they should receive.

This is not just being negative about doctors. I think they really try, that they make a sincere effort to the best of their ability. But given the patient load they have, the pressures they have on them and the way they are schooled, I think that is just their natural outlook. We had to put so much effort and energy in trying to learn the facts, and to cope.

Right from the beginning when we first learned Mom had cancer, and Mom and Dad decided to go to Mexico for three weeks, one of the first things I did was spend days researching. I sought help from someone else in alternative medicine research. We looked world wide. We spent hour after hour trying to dig out this information and getting it through the Internet or having people send the information. It was very hard to come by. There was not much out there. It took a lot of digging to locate it.

Dan also spent a lot of time while Mom and Dad were in Mexico trying to figure out the best doctors, which ones specialized in lung cancer.

DANIEL:

The parent of a man I work with is on a hospital board of trustees. I had him call the head of the medical facility to find out who the best doctors were, and if they were on the up and up. Dad had talked to doctors in Mexico about alternative medicine and having surgery there.

Right or wrong, I was probably one of the biggest advocates for getting Mom back here, getting her under traditional medicine, getting her diagnosed, finding out what the facts were, and then make the decision once we knew what we were dealing with. When she went down there, we still didn't know what she was dealing with.

MICHELE:

We knew she had cancer, but didn't know what caused it.

DANIEL:

We didn't know if it was tied into her back (pain). She had degenerate problems going on in her back. According to the MRI reports, her back was in very bad shape. With my limited knowledge of all the clients I've had with back problems and reading medical records, Mom's back was in really bad shape. That's why I was really concerned when they (Mexico doctors) said they could go in there and fix that. I wanted to find out exactly what we were dealing with, through the proven diagnostic tests, the MRIs, cat scans. Get all that done, then make an intelligent decision what to do. That was my focus.

MICHELE:

While Mom and Dad were gone, I took care of Mother's business office, paid all the bills and ran her business. Dan and I took turns taking care of the house, Dad's mail, all the other things to the extent we could take care of them while they were gone. Although we were working full time, we did that in addition.

When they got back, I spent more time than Dan did, because I was able to take a leave of absence for six weeks. Once I did that, I was spending a minimum of four to six hours a day with Mom. I also was trying to think of things to cook for Dad, and preparing food to take over to the house. I also was looking all over town to learn where we could buy good quality wigs and have people come to the house. She wasn't well enough to go to them, so I was setting up those appointments. I was finding someone to come in to fix up the closet so we could move her clothes into the downstairs bedroom and get the bedroom set up.

When we decided to close down Mom's office, I spent weeks over there. I was going from my work to the office getting boxing, packing, confirming with her to get things where they were supposed to go.

There were quite a few nights I stayed all night with her at the hospital.

My schedule was to go to work, stop at home afterwards and change clothes, go straight to the hospital, stay all night, get up the next morning at 5 o'clock, go home and shower, and go back to work again.

There was a lot that all of us did. Mom's sister-in-law came once or twice a week and did some food preparation. Susan, Dan's wife, came over from time to time. We cleaned the house, tried to do laundry, to help Dad out where we could. Susan's mother brought food, as well as many of the neighbors. So many emotions were involved.

Certainly there has never been a time in my life when I felt that amount of stress and grief. Mom was so totally devastated. When she first came back from Mexico and got all the facts, and they told her what they did, I've never seen anyone in that shape before. It was such a helpless feeling not to know what to do and how to comfort her. And she had a tendency not to come to us, and I'm sure not to burden us.

But when someone came over, like my cousin or aunt, she would just completely fall apart. She would have days on end of being totally despondent. Then she would kind of pick herself up and she'd be okay again. Up to a couple of days before she died, she was saying to me,

"You've got to be positive, Michele. Don't feed into anything negative. Keep positive. Say affirmations for me. Believe it. Visualize."

There were nights when I went home when I just sat and cried for hours by myself. For me, I knew I needed to be strong for her. That's what she needed from me. She needed that support. She didn't need the burden of trying to help me through it. Somewhere God was able to give me the strength to get through it. I only started to break down one time with her. Toward the end. About a week before she died. She got really sick one night. She said, "Don't feed into that". It clicked me out of it, and I was okay until after she died. I never broke down. And I think for her it was important that I could be that strong.

DANIEL:

You were incredibly strong, Michele. I was amazed.

MICHELE:

I need to go back to explain some of my feelings and thoughts. Because of my initial conversations with some of the doctors, my subsequent feelings were perhaps different than they might have been.

Before the meeting after Mom had come back from Mexico, when the lung specialist was going to tell us the results of tests, the type of cancer and what the prognosis was, we had agreed I would talk to the doctor first and discuss the best approach with Mom.

I wanted to talk to him before the whole family sat down. I had wanted to have the conversation with him. But he had put me off, made me wait. Finally he let me come in.

He immediately got very defensive and assumed I was off on my own in doing that. I said, "No, I assure you this has been agreed to by the whole family and I have their support. "

I can be tactful. I have managed people. I know how to deal with a situation like that pretty effectively, normally. I gave it a lot of thought, began with the positive things first, how appreciative we were that he was putting a lot of time and urgency in trying to deal with it for her. But we as a family felt it would help him treat her better if he understood some things about our belief s, philosophies and the kind of person she is.

We talked a little about Dr. Bernie Siegal, an MD who once had cancer, has written several books and lectures on many aspects of medicine. Also, we discussed the fact that Mom was a very positive person and that regardless of what the prognosis was, she needed to be told in a compassionate way that would allow her hope that she had a chance to live a period of time with some quality.

The doctor basically got very angry with me and said, "Frankly I resent the fact you are coming in here and telling me how I should do my job."

He was so insistent I was doing this on my own without anybody else knowing, but I said, "NO-- Dad, Dan and I had discussed it and we were all in agreement."

DANIEL

I remembered talking about it on the telephone. I suggested, "Let's get there early." I think I was with Mom at the time (of the talk).

MICHELE:

He (The doctor) and I went around a little more after that, and I finally said, " Look, I'm not trying to tell you how to do your job, but I have the benefit of forty-some years of knowing and being part of this little family and I know a lot about them that you don't. I think it would help you in terms of how you deal with her."

I told him, "If I were in your shoes, I would welcome that kind of input. If we didn't believe in you, if we didn't have confidence in your ability to deal with this, we wouldn't be here in the first place. We would have gone elsewhere. But I think it's important you understand this about her so you can put it to her in a way that is going to have the most positive possible impact on her."

From that point on, the man was never very friendly with me. But it accomplished the goal, to the extent that when Mom came in and sat down for the meeting - there is no way you can tell someone that (The facts about her condition) and put in a way it would sound good - I felt he handled it about as well as he could.

DANIEL:

He didn't give her a death sentence. But she kept asking, wanting to know, "Is there hope, is there hope?" He may never actually have said "Yes", but he didn't say, "No".

144

MICHELE:

One of the good things was that she could eat anything she wanted. He talked a little about Dr. Bernie Siegel because it came up in the conversation that Mom had read the book and believed in the way he practiced medicine. We talked a little about that, and the fact they went to school together.

I think it helped. One of the things Siegel and others talk a lot about is that the best patients are the ones that give doctors the most trouble, challenge them, don't just accept what they are being told, but ask questions and think about what is best for them and their individual circumstance.

I met with the oncologist several weeks after Mom started the chemo. She was having so much trouble, deathly ill. I was confused. I didn't feel like I understood what was going on, and what was really happening, and where we went from there. I made an appointment and went in to see him myself.

I went through the same type of discussion with him. I asked a lot of questions about her condition, what the chemo could and could not do, what the risks were with it, why do this and not this. It was the same type of discussion as with the lung specialist.

He said, "You have got to face the fact that your mother is dying". I said, "I understand that. I'm not blind. The whole family has understood that from the day she was given the original diagnosis."

But I told him, "We're not a family that's going to roll over and play dead. We are going to do everything we can to make sure she gets the best possible treatment and to make her doctors understand how to deal with her as an individual in the best way to help her through this."

I felt pretty clear about that. I told him point blank, "I understand and I'm accepting that she is going to die. But I do believe that her mental state can have an impact on how long she has, and I'm asking you to try to work with us to help her, not only with the physical but emotionally and mentally."

She was ill at the time, and I went to the hospital and stayed with her. She felt Dad needed to go home and get some rest.

At that point, she said to me, "I'm afraid I'm going to die in the hospital tonight. I'm afraid to be alone."

I said, "I won't leave you. I will stay here with you."

They had a chair in the hospital room. I stayed with her in the chair, and was about three feet away from her. I stayed with her until she fell asleep. Then she had to get up every hour or two at night, and I would get up and help her to the bathroom. That seemed to give her comfort that I was there.

A day or two later, the oncologist came in to see her right after I had left. He woke her up from a sound sleep, flipped on the light. He never came in without at least three or four people with him. I didn't hear this, but she said he told her he was very concerned that the family was not accepting the fact she was dying, and that "it would happen very soon". He added that she was a walking time bomb.

Mom said the oncologist told her he was particularly concerned about me, that I was not accepting, I was in denial, and that she needed to try to make arrangements for me to get grieving counseling.

We knew he had been trying to get her to meet with a psychologist herself, which she was pretty resistant to doing. So he came in, made that pronouncement, and basically gave her the responsibility for dealing with the rest of the family members who he felt were not accepting that she was dying. I was furious about that. The psychiatrist was brought in twice, but Mom resisted.

I understand the doctor was tying to help. He felt she needed psychological support, and they had a person on the staff to provide that. Not to give her hope, but to accept. I also think they were a little afraid of a law suit because of Dan's position. On top of that, there was more than one occasion when an important hospital official personally came to see Mom.

DANIEL:
We had conference calls and the hospital official asked about Mom, I conveyed some problems we were having. He said, "Hey, I'll go in and see. Check on it." When he walks in on one of the hospital floors, and he just doesn't do that, people's ears perk up.

MICHELE:
People talked about that for a long time.

DANIEL:
But it didn't change the methodology.

MICHELE:

It probably did as much harm as it did good, because the doctors resented the fact there was all this involvement and interference.

During that same hospital stay, another morning when I was there with Mom, she wasn't feeling good. She was running a fever. The oncologist came flying in the room sometime between five and six o'clock, and flipped on the light. I had talked to them about that a couple of times, asking, "Can we modify this routine a little, because it's her only quality rest, but when you come in and wake up her up out of a sound sleep, disrupt her rest, throw these things out at her, psychologically its a nightmare. You throw her into this cycle that takes days for her to recover. But nothing changed!

What is so sad is that it was almost impossible for any of us to know what we know now. It was such trauma facing that situation, and learning it so suddenly.

Despite the confusion and apprehensions, and as intimidating as our family might be, even the doctors couldn't help but like Mom. She was a remarkable woman. We always had a strong rapport. But the older I got, the more I realized how strong she was. And I am absolutely amazed that to have gone through this, and even as sick as she was and dying, she had enough concern about the family, and the strength not to want to burden us!

All the emotions she had to be feeling!

I think there are very few people on earth like her that can do that. She is one of the strongest people I've ever known. And I'll always miss her.

* * *

CHAPTER TWENTY-THREE

Information on small-cell lung cancer from the National Cancer Institute
(Reproduced with the permission of the National Cancer Institute)

In attempting to present as much information as possible on small cell lung cancer, I contacted the National Cancer Institute requesting any information they might have on this disease. They were most cooperative and faxed the information which is reproduced in this chapter. At the same time, they gave me permission to reprint the information in this book.

My impression of this contact was that they are very anxious to have patients as well as family and friends contact them for the latest information they have. Of major importance in my estimation is the data they have about clinical trials in progress and will provide this information for specific geographical areas for those who may be interested.

For those who read all of the material including the information in the last 12 pages which is provided to medical providers and doctors, it is not difficult to conclude that small cell lung cancer is for the most part, not curable with the tools and remedies presently approved and available to the medical profession.

Once the disease has begun, my interpretation is that the only hope is that the cancer has not spread and that surgery can remove the infected parts of the lung. Beyond this and short of a miracle, only short term survival and suffering will be experienced as a result of both the cancer and the treatment.

I only wish that I had known that the information that the National Cancer Institute has gathered was available to anyone who asks. And if I had read the material reprinted in this chapter, I would have realized that the disease is a death warrant for the majority of individuals who contract it.

Here then on the pages to follow is the information that the National Cancer Institute faxed to me only a short time after I had spoken with them over the telephone. But unfortunately, all this occurred well after Meryl's death.

* * *

(Cancer Fax from the National Cancer Institute) (301) 402-5874
Information from PDQ _for Patients
(Current as of 02/02/98)

** SMALL CELL LUNG CANCER ** 208/00040

OVERVIEW OF PDQ
_What is **PDQ?** _

PDQ is a computer system that gives up-to-date information on cancer and its prevention, detection, treatment, and supportive care. It is a service of the National Cancer Institute (NCI) for people with cancer and their families and for doctors, nurses, and other health care professionals.

To ensure that it remains current, the information in PDQ is reviewed and updated each month by experts in the fields of cancer treatment, prevention, screening, and supportive care. PDQ also provides information about research on new treatments (clinical trials), doctors who treat cancer, and hospitals with cancer programs. The treatment information in this summary is based on information in the PDQ summary for health professionals on this cancer.

How to use **PDQ** _

PDQ can be used to learn more about current treatment of different kinds of cancer. You may find it helpful to discuss this information with your doctor, who knows you and has the facts about your disease. PDQ can also provide the names of additional health care professionals who specialize in treating patients with cancer.

Before you start treatment, you also may want to think about taking part in a clinical trial. PDQ can be used to learn more about these trials. A clinical trial is a research study that attempts to improve current treatments or finds information on new treatments for patients with cancer. Clinical trials are based on past studies and information discovered in the laboratory. Each trial answers certain scientific questions in order to find new and better ways to help patients with cancer. Information is collected about new treatments, their risks, andhow well they do or do not work. When clinical trials show that a new treatment is better than the treatment currently used as 'standard" treatment, the new treatment may become the standard treatment. Listings of current clinical trials are available on PDQ. Many cancer doctors who take part in clinical trials are listed in PDQ.

To learn more about cancer and how it is treated, or to learn more about clinical trials for your kind of cancer, call the National Cancer Institutes Cancer Information Service. The number is 1-800-4-CANCER (1-800-422-6237); TTY at *1-800-332-8615*. The call is free and a trained information specialist will be available to answer cancer-related questions.

PDQ is updated whenever there is new information. Check with the Cancer Information Service to be sure that you have the most up-to-date information.

** DESCRIPTION **
--What is small cell lung cancer? _

Small cell lung cancer is a disease in which cancer (malignant) cells are found in the tissues of the lungs. The lungs are a pair of cone-shaped organs that take up much of the inside of the chest. The lungs bring oxygen into the body and take out carbon dioxide. which is a waste product of the body's cells. Tubes called bronchi make up the inside of the lungs.

There are two kinds of lung cancer based on how the cells look under a microscope: small cell and non-small cell. If you have non-small cell lung cancer, see the PDQ patient information statement on non-small cell lung cancer.

Small cell lung cancer is usually found in people who smoke or who used to smoke cigarettes. You should see your doctor if you have any of the following problems: a cough or chest pain that doesn't go away, a wheezing sound in your breathing, shortness of breath, coughing up blood, hoarseness, or swelling in your face and neck.

If you have symptoms, your doctor may want to look into the bronchi through a special instrument, called a bronchoscope, that slides down the throat and into the bronchi. This test, called bronchoscopy, is usually done in the hospital. Before the test, you will be given a local anesthetic (a drug that makes you lose feeling for a short period of time) in the back of your throat. You may feel some pressure, but you usually do not feel pain. Your doctor can take cells from the walls of the bronchi tubes or cut small pieces of tissue to look at under the microscope to see if there are any cancer cells. This is called a biopsy.

Your doctor may also use a needle to remove tissue from a place in the lung that may be hard to reach with the bronchoscope. A cut will be made in your skin and the needle will be put in between your ribs. This is called a needle aspiration biopsy. Your doctor will look at the tissue under the microscope to see if there are any cancer cells. Before the test, you will be given a local anesthetic to keep you from feeling pain.

Your chance of recovery (prognosis) and choice of treatment depend on the stage of the cancer (whether it• is just in the lung or has spread to other places), gender, and general state of health.

** STAGE EXPLANATION **

-Stages of small cell lung cancer -

Once small cell lung cancer has been found, more tests will be done to find out if cancer cells have spread from one or both lungs to other parts of the body (staging). Your doctor needs to know the stage of your disease to plan treatment. The following stages are used for small cell lung cancer:

-Limited stage -

Cancer is found only in one lung and in nearby lymph nodes. (Lymph nodes are small, bean-shaped structures that are found throughout the body. They produce and store infection-fighting cells.)

-Extensive stage -

Cancer has spread outside of the lung where it began to other tissues in the chest or to other parts of the body.

-Recurrent stage -

Recurrent disease means that the cancer has come back (recurred) after it has been treated. It may come back in the lungs or in another part of the body.

** TREATMENT OPTION OVERVIEW**

- How small cell lung cancer is treated -

There are treatments for all patients with small cell lung cancer. Three kinds of treatment are used:

Surgery (taking out the cancer)

Radiation therapy (using high-dose x-rays or other high-energy rays to kill cancer cells

Chemotherapy (using drugs to kill cancer cells).

Additionally, clinical trials are testing the effect of new therapies on the treatment of small cell lung cancer.

Surgery may be used if the cancer is found only in one lung and in nearby lymph nodes. Because this type of lung cancer is usually not found in only one lung, surgery alone is not often used. Occasionally, surgery may be used to help determine exactly which type of lung cancer you have. If you do have surgery, your doctor may take out the cancer in one of the following operations:

Wedge resection removes only a small part of the lung.

Lobectomy removes an entire section (lobe) of the lung.

Pneumonectomy removes the entire lung.

During surgery, your doctor will also take out lymph nodes to see if they contain cancer.

Radiation therapy uses x-rays or other high-energy rays to kill cancer cells and shrink tumors. Radiation therapy for small cell lung cancer usually comes from a machine outside the body (external beam radiation therapy). It may be used to kill cancer cells in the lungs or in other parts of the body where the cancer has spread. Radiation therapy may also be used to prevent the cancer from growing in the brain. This is called prophylactic cranial irradiation (PCI). Because PCI may affect your brain functions, your doctor will help you decide whether to have this kind of radiation therapy. Radiation therapy can be used alone or in addition to surgery and/or chemotherapy.

Chemotherapy is the most common treatment for all stages of small cell lung cancer. Chemotherapy may be taken by pill, or it may be put into the body by a needle in the vein or muscle. Chemotherapy is called a systemic treatment because the drug enters the bloodstream, travels through the body, and can kill cancer cells outside the lungs, including cancer cells that have spread to the brain.

_Treatment by stage _

Treatment for small cell lung cancer depends on the stage of the disease, your age, and your overall condition.

You may receive treatment that is considered standard based on its effectiveness in a number of patients in past studies, or you may choose to go into a clinical trial. Most patients are not cured with standard therapy and some standard treatments may have more side effects than are desired. For these reasons, clinical trials are designed to find better ways to treat cancer patients and are based on the most up-to-date information. Clinical trials are going on in most parts of the country for most stages of small cell lung cancer. If wish to know more about clinical trials, call the:

Cancer Information Service **at 1-800-4-CANCER (1-800-422-**6237); **TTY at 1-800-332-8615.**

** LIMITED STAGE SMALL CELL LUNG CANCER **

Your treatment may be one of the following:
1. Chemotherapy and radiation therapy to the chest with or without radiation therapy to the brain to prevent spread of the cancer (prophytlacticcrainial irradiation.
2. Chemotherapy with or without prophylactic cranial irradiation.
3. Surgery followed by chemotherapy with or without prophylactic cranial irradiation.

Clinical trials are testing new drugs and new ways of giving all of the above treatments.

EXTENSIVE STAGE SMALL CELL LUNG CANCER

Your treatment may be one of the following:
1. Chemotherapy with or without radiation therapy to the brain to prevent spread of the cancer (prophylactic cranial irradiation).

2. Radiation therapy to places in the body where the cancer spread, such as the brain, one, or spine to relieve symptoms.

Clinical trials are testing new drugs and new ways of giving all of the above treatments.

·· RECURRENT SMALL CELL LUNG CANCER ··

Your treatment may be one of the following:

1. Radiation therapy to reduce discomfort.
2. A clinical trial testing new drugs.

**TO LEARN MORE ··   CALL 1-800-4-CANCER

To learn more about small cell lung cancer, call the National Cancer Institute's Cancer Information Service at 1-800-4-CANCER (1-800-422-6237): TTY at 1-800-332-8615. By dialing this toll-free number, you can speak with someone who can answer your questions.

The Cancer Information Service can also send you booklets. The following booklets about lung cancer may be helpful to you:

What You Need To Know About Lung Cancer
Research Report: Cancer of the Lung

The following general booklets on questions related to cancer may also be helpful:

What You Need To Know About Cancer
Taking Time: Support for People with Cancer and the People Who Care About Them
What Are Clinical Trials All About?
Chemotherapy and You: A Guide to Self-Help During Treatment
Radiation Therapy and You: A Guide to Self-Help During Treatment
Eating Hints for Cancer Patients
Advanced Cancer: Living Each Day
When Cancer Recurs: Meeting the Challenge Again

There are other places where you can get material about cancer treatment and information about services to help you. You can check the social service office at your hospital for local and national agencies that help with your finances, getting to and from treatment, care at home, and dealing with your problems.

You can also write to the National Cancer Institute at this address:

National Cancer Institute
Office of Cancer Communications
31 Center Drive, MSC 2580
Bethesda, MD 20892-25 80

This information from PDQ is reviewed regularly by members of the PDQ Editorial Boards. If you have specific comments on the content of this information, direct them to: PDQ Editorial Board, ICIC/NCI, 903001d Georgetown Rd, Bethesda, MD 20892-2650, fax: 301-480-8105.Comments will be forwarded to the Editorial Board for review.

If you want to know more about cancer and how it is treated, or if you wish to learn about clinical trials for your kind of cancer, you can call the NCI's Cancer Information Service at 1-800-422-6237, toll free.

****

This information is intended for use by doctors and other health care professionals. If you are a cancer patient, your doctor can explain how it applies to you. or you can call the Cancer Information Service at 1-8004226237. Cancer Fax also contains information from PDQ for patients. See the Cancer Fax Contents List for more information.

****

Information from PDQ -- for Health Professionals
**   Small cell lung cancer **   208/00040

**   PROGNOSIS **

Without treatment, small cell carcinoma of the lung has the most aggressive clinical course of any type of pulmonary tumor, with median survival from diagnosis of only 2-4 months. Compared with other cell types of lung cancer. small cell carcinoma has a greater tendency to be widely disseminated by the time of diagnosis, but is much more responsive to chemotherapy and irradiation.

Because of its propensity for distant metastases, localized forms of treatment such as surgical resection or radiotherapy, rarely produce long-term survival [1]. With incorporation of current chemotherapy regimens into the treatment program, however, survival is unequivocally prolonged, with at least a 4 to 5-fold improvement in median survival compared with patients who are given no therapy. Furthermore, about 10% of the total population of patients remain free of disease over two years from the start of therapy, the time period during which most relapses occur. However, even these patients are at risk of dying from lung cancer (both small and non-small cell types). [2] The overall survival at 5 years is less than 5%.

At the time of diagnosis, approximately one-third of patients with small cell carcinoma will have tumor confined to the hemithorax of origin, the mediastinum, or the supraclavicular lymph nodes. These patients are designated as having limited stage disease, and most 2-year disease-free survivors come from this group. In limited stage disease, median survival of 10-16 months with current forms of treatment can reasonably be expected. A small proportion of patients with limited stage disease may benefit from surgery with or without adjuvant chemotherapy; these patients have an even better prognosis. Patients with tumor that has spread beyond the supraclavicular areas are said to have extensive stage disease and have a worse prognosis than patients with limited stage. Median survival of 6-12 months is reported with currently available therapy, but long-term disease-free survival is rare. Patients who achieve complete response to treatment have the best overall survival. [3]

Some retrospective studies have shown that young women appear to have a more favorable prognosis. [4] Furthermore. in both limited and extensive stage disease, performance status is an extremely important prognostic factor.[5,6] In a large retrospective analysis of 1,714 patients treated with various combination chemotherapy regimens, the 5-year survival rate was 3.5%.[6] In general, patients who are confined to bed tolerate aggressive forms of treatment poorly, have increased morbidity, and rarely attain 2-year disease-free survival. However, patients with poor performance status can often derive significant palliative benefit and prolongation of survival from treatment.

Regardless of stage, the current prognosis for patients with small cell lung cancer is unsatisfactory, even though considerable improvements in diagnosis and therapy have been made over the past 10-15 years. Therefore, all patients with this type of cancer may appropriately be considered for inclusion in clinical trials at the time of diagnosis.

References:

1 Prasad US, Naylor AR, Walker WS, et al. : Long-term survival after pulmonary resection for small cell carcinoma of the lung. Thorax 44(10)784-787, 1989.

2. Johnson BE, Grayson J, Makuch RW, et al: ten-year survival of patients with small-cell. lung cancer treated with combination chemotherapy with or without irradiation, Journal of Clinical Oncology 8(3): 396-401, 1990.

3. Perry MC, Eaton WL, Propert KJ, et al: Chemotherapy with or without radiation therapy in limited small-cell carcinoma of the lung. New England Journal of Medicine 316(15): 912-918. 1987.

4. Wolf M. Holle R, Hans K, et al. : Analysis of prognostic factors in 766 patients with small cell lung cancer (SCLC): the role of sex as a

predictor for survival. British Journal of Cancer 63(6): 986-992. 1991.

5. Rawson NS, Peto J: An overview of prognostic actors in small cell lung cancer: a report from the subcommittee for the management of lung cancer of the United Kingdom Coordinating Committee on Cancer Research. British Journal of Cancer 61(4): 597-604, 1990.

6. Lassen U, Osterlind K, Hansen M, et al. : Long-term survival in small-cell lung cancer: post treatment characteristics in patients surviving 5 to 18+years - an analysis of 1,714 consecutive patients. Journal of Clinical Oncology 13(5): **1215-1220 1995.**

** CELLULAR CLASSIFICATION **

Review of pathologic material by an experienced lung cancer pathologist is critical prior to initiating treatment for any patient with small cell lung cancer, since the intermediate subtype of small cell carcinoma and the more readily recognized lymphocyte-like or 'oat cell subtype are equally responsive to treatment,

The current classification of subtypes of small cell lung cancer are:

[l] Oat cell intermediate mixed (small cell combined with other cell types of lung {carcinoma) There is increasing evidence that light microscopy has some limitations as a means of classifying bronchogenic carcinomas, particularly small cell carcinomas. Electron microscopy. which can detect neuroendocrine granules. may help to differentiate between small cell and non-small cell cancers.[2]

Neuroendocrine carcinomas of the lung represent a spectrum of disease. At one extreme is small cell lung cancer, which has a poor prognosis. At the other extreme are bronchial carcinoids. with an excellent prognosis after surgical excision.[3] Between these extremes is an unusual entity called well-differentiated neuroendocrine carcinoma of the lung.[4] It has been referred to as malignant carcinoid, metastasizing bronchial adenoma, pleomorphic carcinoid, nonbenign carcinoid tumor, and atypical carcinoid. Like small cell lung cancer. it occurs primarily in cigarette smokers, but it metastasizes less frequently. The 5-year survival rate is greater than 50% in some series, and surgical cure appears possible in most stage I patients. Careful diagnosis is important, however, since the differential pathologic diagnosis from small cell lung cancer may be difficult.

References:

1. Kreyberg L, Liebow AA, Uehlinger EA: International Histologic

Classification of Tumours: No. 1. Histological Typing of Lung Tumours, Geneva World Health Organization. 2nd ed.. 1981.

2. Mooi IJJ, Van Zandwijk N, Dingemans KP. et al, The 'Grey Area between small cell and non-small cell lung carcinomas: light and electron microscopy versus clinical data in 14 cases. Journal of Pathology 149(1): 49-54, 1986.

3. Harpole DH. Feldman JM, Buchanan 5, et al. Bronchial carcinoid tumors: are retrospective analysis of 126 patients. Annals of Thoracic Surgery 54(1): 50-55, 1992.

4. Lequaglie C. Patriarca C. Cataldo I, et al. : Prognosis of resected well-differentiated neuroendocrine carcinoma of the lung. Chest 100(4): 1053-1056. 1991.

** STAGE INFORMATION **

Staging procedures do not currently have a major impact on treatment for small cell lung cancer since patients should initially receive combination chemotherapy regardless of the extent of tumor dissemination. However. determining the stage of cancer by non-surgical means allows a better assessment of prognosis and identifies sites of tumor that can be evaluated for response. In clinical situations where the choice of treatment is affected by stage, particularly when chest irradiation or surgical excision is added to chemotherapy alone for limited stage patients, results of the staging process have therapeutic implications. Staging procedures commonly used to document distant metastases include bone marrow examination computed tomographic or radionuclide scans of brain and liver, and radionuclide bone scans.

Because occult or overt metastatic disease is present at diagnosis in most patients survival is usually not affected by small differences in the amount of locoregional tumor involvement, Therefore, the detailed TNM staging system developed for lung cancer by the American Joint Committee on Cancer (AJCC) is not commonly employed in patients with small cell carcinoma. A simple 2-stage system developed by the Veterans Administration Lung Cancer Study Group is most commonly used. [1}

The recently published international staging system, which is outlined in detail in the PDQ state-of-the-art statement for non-small cell lung cancer, may also be utilized, particularly for the small minority of patients who may be candidates for surgical resection. [2]

-- Limited stage --

Limited stage small cell lung cancer means tumor confined to the hemithorax of origin, the mediastinum, and the supraclavicular nodes, which is encompassable within a "tolerable' radiotherapy port. There is no universally accepted definition of this term, and patients with pleural effusion, massive or multiple ipsilateral pulmonary tumor. and contralateral supraclavicular nodes have been both included within and excluded from limited stage by various groups.

-- Extensive stage

Extensive stage small cell lung cancer means tumor that is too widespread to be included within the definition of limited stage disease.[1,2]

References:
1. Zelen M: Keynote address on biostatistics and data retrieval. Cancer Chemotherapy Reports 4(2): 31-42. 1973.
2. Mountain CF: A new international staging system for lung cancer. Chest 89 (Suppl 4): 225-233, 1986

** TREATMENT OPTION OVERVIEW **

In small cell lung cancer, the majority of patients die of their tumor despite state-of-the-art treatment. Most of the improvements in survival in small cell lung cancer are attributable to clinical, trials which have attempted to improve upon the best available, accepted therapy. Patient entry into such studies is highly desirable,

Areas of active clinical evaluation in small cell lung cancer include drug regimens composed of standard and new agents, variation of drug doses in current regimens, and study of the possible benefits of adding surgical resection of the primary tumor or radiotherapy to the chest and other sites to combination chemotherapy. Controversy exists over the issue of whether increasing the dose rate of commonly used front-line regimens above levels that produce modest toxicity will produce improved survival. Retrospective studies are plagued by methodologic difficulties and show inconsistent results.[1] The issue is best settled by randomized trials. A prospective randomized study in extensive stage disease does not suggest any advantage to increasing the standard doses of etoposide plus cisplatin.[2] Even chemotherapy of the intensity used in autologous bone marrow transplant regimens has not clearly been shown to improve survival in patients with small cell lung cancer. [3,4]

The designations in PDQ that treatments are "standard" or "under clinical evaluation" are not to be used as a basis for reimbursement determinations.

References:

1. Klasa RJ, Murray N, Coldman AJ: Dose-intensity meta-analysis of chemotherapy regimens in small-cell carcinoma of the lung. Journal of Clinical Oncology 9(3): 499-508, 1991.
2. Ihde DC, Mulshine JL, Kramer BS, et al. : Prospective randomized comparison of high-dose and standard-dose etoposide and cisplatin chemotherapy in patients with extensive-stage small-cell lung cancer. Journal of Clinical Oncology 12(10): 2022-2034, 1994.
3. Ihde DC. Deisseroth AB, Lichter AS. et al. : Late intensive combined modality therapy followed by autologous bone marrow infusion in extensive-stage small-cell lung cancer. Journal of Clinical Oncology 4(10): 1443-1454, 1986.
4. Humblet Y, Symann M, Bosly A. et al. : Late intensification chemotherapy with autologous bone marrow transplantation in selected small-cell carcinoma of the lung: a randomized study. Journal of Clinical Oncology 5(12): 1864-1873. 1987.

** LIMITED STAGE SMALL CELL LUNG CANCER **

In patients with small cell lung cancer. combination chemotherapy produces results that are clearly superior to single-agent treatment, and moderately intensive doses of drugs are superior to doses that produce only minimal or mild hematologic toxicity. Current programs yield overall objective response rates of 65%-90% and complete response rates of 45%-75%. Because of the frequent presence of occult metastatic disease, chemotherapy is the cornerstone of treatment for limited stage small cell lung cancer. Combinations containing two or more drugs are needed for maximal effect.

The relative effectiveness of many 2- to 4-drug combination programs appears similar, and a large number of combinations have been used. Therefore, a representative selection of regimens that have been found to be effective by at least two independent groups has been provided below. The use of alternating chemotherapy regimens has not proven more effective than etoposide plus cisplatin.[1-3] Optimal duration of chemotherapy is not clearly defined, but there is no obvious improvement in survival when the duration of drug administration exceeds 4-6 months. There is no evidence from randomized clinical trials that maintenance chemotherapy is of benefit. [2. 4.5]

Mature results of prospective randomized trials suggest that combined modality therapy produces a modest but significant improvement in survival compared with chemotherapy alone. Two meta-analyses showed an improvement in 3-year survival rates of about 5% for those receiving chemotherapy and radiotherapy compared to those receiving chemotherapy alone.[6.7] Most of the benefit occurred in patients less than 65 years of age. Combined modality treatment is associated with increased morbidity and, in some trials, increased treatment-related mortality from pulmonary and hematologic toxic effects; proper administration requires close collaboration between medical and radiation oncologists. [8, 9] In general, those studies showing a positive effect for combined modality therapy employed thoracic irradiation early in the course of treatment. [9]

Studies strongly suggest that minimal tumor doses in the range of 5000 cGy or more (standard fractionation) are necessary to effectively control tumors in the thorax.

Patients presenting with superior vena cava syndrome are treated with combination chemotherapy with or without radiation therapy. A small minority of limited stage patients with adequate pulmonary function and with tumor pathologically confined to the lung of origin, or the lung and ipsilateral hilar lymph nodes, may possibly benefit from surgical resection with or without adjuvant chemotherapy. [10-12]

Because of the high frequency of development of brain metastases in small cell carcinoma, particularly in patients with prolonged survival, prophylactic cranial irradiation (PCI) has been administered by many physicians. Prospective studies have shown that PCI reduces the frequency of clinically detected brain metastases, particularly in patients with a complete response to therapy, but have not shown improvement in overall survival. There are increasing reports of significant neurologic, mental, and psychometric deficits in long-term survivors treated with PCI, and the optimal dose and schedule of PCI has not been defined.[13,14] A review of 7 studies in which PCI was employed reveals that in 96 long-term survivors, neuropsychologic impairment was noted in 76% of examined patients, whereas in a group of 20 long-term survivors not treated with PCI, only 15% had neuropsychologic impairment.[15] An international trial is being performed to assess the effect of PCI in patients who achieve a complete response. Neurotoxicity associated with PCI may be exacerbated by various chemotherapeutic agents. Experience has demonstrated that lomustine and PCI are associated with a 17% incidence of neurotoxicity.[16] Other chemotherapy agents may also increase the incidence of neurotoxicity in patients receiving cranial irradiation. PCI cannot be routinely recommended for patients with small cell lung cancer: clinical benefit is likely only in those who achieve complete remission and experience long-term survival. Potential risks and benefits should be carefully considered and discussed with the patient before employing PCI in this disease. [15]

Treatment options:
Standard:
1. Combination chemotherapy with one of the following regimens and chest irradiation (with or without PCI given to patients with complete responses):

The following regimens produce similar survival outcomes:
EP or EC: etoposide + cisplatin or carboplatin [17. 18]CAV: cyclophosphamide + doxorubicin + vincristine [19] CAE: cyclophosphamide + doxorubicin + etoposide [20] ICE: ifosfamide + carboplatin + etoposide [21]

Other regimens appear to produce similar survival outcomes but have been studied less extensively or are in less common use including: yclophosphamide + methotrexate + lomustine + vincristine [23] cyclophosphamide + doxorubicin + etoposide + vincristine [24] CEV: cyclophosphamide + etoposide + vincristine [25] oral etoposide. [26]

2. Combination chemotherapy (with or without PCI in patients with complete responses), especially in patients with impaired pulmonary function or poor performance status.

3. Surgical resection of pulmonary tumor in highly selected cases. followed by combination chemotherapy with or without PCI. [27,28]

Under clinical evaluation:

Areas of active clinical evaluation in small cell lung cancer include new drug regimens composed of standard and new agents, variation of drug doses in current regimens, surgical resection of the primary tumor or radiotherapy to the chest and other sites added to combination chemotherapy. new radiotherapy schedules, and timing of thoracic radiation that may allow improved tumor control with less toxicity. [8,29.30]

References:

1. Einhorn LH, Crawford J, Birch R, et al. : Cisplatin plus etoposide consolidation following cyclophosphamide, doxorubicin, and vincristine in limited small-cell lung cancer. Journal of Clinical Oncology 6(3): '451-456, 1988

2. Giaccone G. Dalesio 0, McVie GJ. et al. : Maintenance chemotherapy in small-cell lung cancer: long-term results of a randomized trial. Journal of Clinical Oncology 11(7): 1230-1240, 1993.

3. Wolf M. Pritsch M. Drings P, et al. : Cyclic-alternating versus response-oriented chemotherapy in small-cell lung cancer: a German multicenter randomized trial of 321 patients. Journal of Clinical Oncology 9(4): 614-624, 1991.

4. Spiro SG. Souhami RL, Geddes DM, et al. : Duration of chemotherapy in small cell lung cancer: a Cancer Research Campaign trial. British Journal of Cancer 59(4): 578-583, 1989.

5. Bleehen NM, Fayers PM, Girling DJ, et al.: Controlled trial of twelve versus six courses of chemotherapy in the treatment of small-cell lung cancer: report to the Medical Research Council by its Lung Cancer Working Party. British Journal of Cancer 59(4): 584-590, 1989.

6. Pignon JP, Arriagada R, Ihde DC. et al. : A meta-analysis of thoracic radiotherapy for small-cell lung cancer. New England Journal of Medicine 327(23): 1618-1624, 1992.

7. Warde P Payne D: Does thoracic irradiation improve survival and local control in limited-stage small-cell carcinoma of the lung? A meta-analysis. Journal of Clinical Oncology 10(6): 890-895, 1992.

8. Turrisi AT: Incorporation of radiotherapy fractionation in the combined-modality treatment of limited small-cell lung cancer. Chest 103(4, Suppl): 418s-422s, 1993.

9. Murray N, Coy P, Pater JL, et al. : Importance of timing for thoracic irradiation in the combined modality treatment of limited-stage small-cell lung cancer. Journal of Clinical Oncology 11(2): 336-344, 1993

10. Osterlind K, Hansen M, Hansen HH, et al.: Treatment policy of surgery in small cell carcinoma of the lung: retrospective analysis of a series of 874 consecutive patients. Thorax 40(4): 272-277, 1985.

11. Shepherd FA, Ginsberg RJ, Patterson GA, et al.: A prospective study of adjuvant surgical resection after chemotherapy for limited small cell lung cancer: a University of Toronto Lung Oncology Group study. Journal of Thoracic and Cardiovascular Surgery 97(2): 177-186, 1989.

12. Prasad US, Naylor AR, Walker WS, et al. : Long-term survival after pulmonary resection for small cell carcinoma of the lung. Thorax '-P4(10): 78L4~787. 1989.

13. Harris DT: Prophylactic cranial irradiation in small-cell lung cancer. Seminars in Oncology 20(4): 338-350. 1993.

14. Crossen JR Garwood D, Glatstein E, et al.: Neurobehavioral sequelac of cranial irradiation in adults: a review of radiation-induced encephalopathy. Journal of Clinical Oncology 12(3): 627-642 1994.

15. Ihde DC: Prophylactic cranial irradiation: current controversies. Lung Cancer 9(Suppl 1): s69-s74, 1993.

16. Frytak 5, Shaw JN, O'Neill BP. et al. : Leukoencephalopathy in small cell lung cancer patients receiving prophylactic cranial irradiation. American Journal of Clinical Oncology 12(1): 27-33, 1989.

17. Evans UK, Shepherd FA, Feld R, et al.: VP-16 and cisplatin as first-line therapy for small--cell lung cancer. Journal of Clinical Oncology 3(11):1471-1477, 1985.

18. Skarlos DV, Samantas E, Kosmidis P et al. : Randomized comparison of etoposide-cisplatin vs. etoposide-carboplatin and irradiation in small-cell lung cancer: a Helienic Co-operative Oncology Group study. Annals of Oncology 5(7): 601-607, 1994.

19. Greco FA, Richardson RL, Snell JD, et al.: Small cell lung cancer: complete remission and improved survival, American Journal of Medicine 66(4): 625-630, 1979.

20. Aisner J, Whitacre M, Van Echo DA, et al. : Combination chemotherapy for small cell carcinoma of the lung: continuous versus alternating non-cross-resistant comb mat ions. Cancer Treatment Reports 66(2): 221-230, 1982.

21. Thatcher N: Ifosfamide/carboplatin/etoposide (ICE) regimen in small cell lung cancer. Lung Cancer 9(Suppi 1): sSI-s67. 1993.

22. Cohen MH, Creaven PJ. Fossieck BE, et al. : Intensive chemotherapy of small cell bronchogenic carcinoma. Cancer Treatment Reports 61(3): 349-354, 1977.

23. Hansen HH, Dombernowsky P, Hansen M, et al. : Chemotherapy of advanced small-cell anaplastic carcinoma: superiority of a four-drug combination to a three-drug combination. Annals of Internal Medicine 89(2): 177-181, 1978.

24. Eagan RT. Frytak 5, Fleming TR. et al. : An evaluation of low-dose cisplatin as part of combined modality therapy of limited small cell lung cancer. Cancer Clinical Trials 4(3): 267-271. 1981.

25. Hong WK, Nicaise C, Lawson R, et al.: Etoposide combined with cyclophosphamide plus vincristine compared with doxorubicin plus cyclophosphamide plus vincristine and with high-dose cyclophosphamide plus vincristine in the treatment of small-cell carcinoma of the lung: a randomized trial of the Bristol Lung Cancer Study Group. Journal of Clinical Oncology 7(4): 450-456, 1989.

26. Carney DN, Keane M, Grogan L: Oral etoposide in small cell lung cancer. Seminars in Oncology 19(6, Suppl 14): 40-44, 1992.

27. Maassen U. Greschuchna D, Martinez I: The role of surgery in the treatment of small cell carcinoma of the lung. Recent Results in Cancer Research 97: 107-115, 1985.

28. Baker RR, Ettinger DS, Ruckdeschel JD, et al. : The role of surgery in the management of selected patients with small-cell carcinoma of the lung. Journal of Clinical Oncology 5(5): 697-702, 1987.

29. Ihde DC, Grayson J, Woods E, et al. : Twice daily chest irradiation as an adjuvant to etoposide/cisplatin therapy of limited stage small cell lung cancer. In: Salmon SE, Ed. : Adjuvant Therapy of Cancer VI. Philadelphia: UB. Saunders Company. 1990. pp 162-165.

30. Armstrong JG, Rosenstein MM, Kris MG, et al. : Twice daily thoracic irradiation for limited small cell lung cancer. International Journal of Radiation Oncology. Biology, Physics 21(5): 1269-1274. 1991.

** EXTENSIVE STAGE SMALL CELL LUNG CANCER **

As in limited stage small cell carcinoma, chemotherapy should be given as multiple agents in doses associated with at least moderate toxicity in order to produce the best results in extensive stage disease. Doses and schedules used in current programs yield overall response rates of 70%-85% and complete response rates of 20%-30% in extensive stage disease. Since overt disseminated disease is present. combination chemotherapy is the cornerstone of treatment for this stage of small cell lung cancer. Combinations containing two or more drugs are needed for maximal benefit.

The relative effectiveness of many 2- to 4-drug combination programs appears similar. and there are a large number of potential combinations. Therefore. a representative selection of regimens that have been found to be effective by at least two independent groups has been provided. Some physicians have administered two of these or other regimens in alternating sequences, but there is no proof that this strategy yields substantial survival improvement.[l-3] Optimal duration of chemotherapy is not clearly defined, but there is no obvious improvement in survival when the duration of drug administration exceeds 6 months. [4] There is no clear evidence from reported data that maintenance chemotherapy is of benefit. [5-7]

Combination chemotherapy plus chest irradiation does not appear to improve survival compared with chemotherapy alone in extensive stage small cell lung cancer. However, radiotherapy plays an extremely important role in palliation of symptoms of the primary tumor and of metastatic disease. particularly brain, epidural. and bone metastases.

Chest irradiation is sometimes given for superior vena cava syndrome, but chemotherapy alone (with irradiation reserved for non-responding patients) is appropriate initial treatment. Brain metastases are often treated with whole-brain radiotherapy. However, intracranial metastases from small cell carcinoma appear to respond to chemotherapy as readily as other metastatic locations. [8]

Because of the increasing likelihood of development of brain metastases with more prolonged survival, prophylactic cranial irradiation (PCI) is sometimes administered to extensive stage small cell lung cancer patients, particularly those with a complete response to therapy. However, PCI has not been shown to improve survival. (9, 10] Because of increasing reports on significant neurological, mental, and psychometric deficits in long-term survivors treated with high daily dose fractionation of irradiation to the brain (300 cGy or greater), such high dose daily fractions should be avoided. [11]

Many more patients with extensive stage small cell carcinoma have greatly impaired performance status at the time of diagnosis when compared to patients with limited stage disease. Such patients have a poor prognosis and tolerate aggressive chemotherapy or combined modality therapy poorly and may be managed with less intensive treatment. However, even these patients derive survival benefit from chemotherapy. Single-agent etoposide or oral etoposide combined with other active drugs are appropriate therapies for these patients. [12-14]

TREATMENT OPTIONS:

STANDARD:
1. Combination chemotherapy with one of the following regimens with or without PCI:
    The following regimens produce similar survival outcomes:
    CAV: cyclophosphamide + doxorubicin + vincristine [15,16]
    CAE: cyclophosphamide + doxorubicin + etoposide [17]
    EP or EC: etoposide + cisplatin or carboplatin [18, 19]
       ICE: ifosfamide + carboplatin + etoposide [20]
    Other regimens appear to produce similar survival outcomes but have been studied less extensively or are in less common use, including:
    cyclophosphamide + methotrexate + lomustine [21]
    cyclophosphamide + methotrexate + lomustine + vincristine [22]
    cyclophosphamide + doxorubicin + etoposide + vincristine [23]
    CEV: cyclophosphamide + etoposide + vincristine [24]
    single-agent etoposide or teniposide [12, 13]
2. Combination chemotherapy and chest irradiation with or without PCI.
3. Radiotherapy to sites of metastatic disease unlikely to be immediately palliated by chemotherapy, especially brain, epidural, and bone metastases.
4. Identification of effective new agents is difficult in patients who have previously been treated with standard chemotherapy because response rates to agents, even of known efficacy, are known to be lower than in previously untreated patients. This situation led to the suggestion that patients with extensive disease who are medically stable to be treated with new agents under evaluation, with provisions for early change to standard combination therapy if there is no response [25] Such a strategy has been shown to be feasible, with survival comparable to survival with initial standard therapy, as long as the patients with extensive disease are carefully chosen. [26-28] Nevertheless, this strategy is a controversial one.

[29] A variety of either strategies have been proposed depending upon the activity of the new agent in other tumors, in preclinical small cell lung cancer models, or the activity of drug analogs. [30] Two active single agents undergoing further evaluation include teniposide and paclitaxel [12,31]

UNDER CLINICAL EVALUATION:
Areas of active clinical evaluation in small cell lung cancer include new drug regimens composed of standard and new agents, variation of drug doses in current regimens, and study of the possible benefits of adding radiotherapy to the chest and other sites to combination chemotherapy

1. Evans UK, Feld R. Murray N, et al.: Superiority of alternating non-cross resistant chemotherapy in extensive small cell lung cancer. Annals of Internal Medicine 107(4): 451-458, 1987

2. Wolf M, Pritsch M, Drings P, et al. : Cyclic-alternating versus response -oriented chemotherapy in small-cell lung cancer: a German multicenter randomized trial of 321 patients. Journal of Clinical oncology 9(4): 614-624, 1991,

3. Roth BJ. Johnson DH, Schacter LP, et al.: Randomized study of cyclophosphamide, doxorubicin, and vincristine versus etoposide and cisplatin versus alternation of these two regimens in extensive small-cell lung cancer: a phase III trial of the Southeastern Cancer Study Group. Journal of Clinical Oncology 10(2): 282-291. 1992.

4. Spiro SG, Souhami RL. Geddes DM. et al. : Duration of chemotherapy in small cell lung cancer: a Cancer Research Campaign trial. British Journal of Cancer 59(4): 578-583, 1989.

5. Giaccone G, Dalesio 0, McVie GJ, et al. : Maintenance chemotherapy in small-cell lung cancer: long-term results of a randomized trial. Journal of Clinical Oncology 11(7): 1230-1240. 1993.

6. Bleehen NM, Fayers PM, Girling DJ, et al. : Controlled trial of twelve versus six courses of chemotherapy in the treatment of small-cell lung cancer: report to the Medical Research Council by its Lung Cancer Working Party. British Journal of Cancer 59(4): 584-590, 1989.

7. Greco FA: Treatment options for patients with relapsed small cell lung cancer. Lung Cancer 9(Suppl 1): s85-s89, 1993.

8. Shepherd FA, Evans WK, MacCormick R, et al: Cyclophosphamide, doxorubicin, and vincristine in etoposide and cisplatin-resistant small cell lung cancer. Cancer Treatment Reports 71(10): 941-944, 1987

9. Harris DT: Prophylactic cranial irradiation in small cell lung cancer Seminars in Oncology 20(4): 338-350, 1993

10. Ihde DC: Prophylactic cranial irradiation: current controversies. Lung Cancer 9(Suppl 1): s69-s74, 1993.

11. Crossen JR. Garwood D, Glatstein E, et al. : Neurobehavioral sequelae of cranial irradiation in adults: a review of radiation-induced encephalopathy. Journal of Clinical Oncology 12(3): 627-642, 1994.

12. Bork E, Ersboll J, Dombernowsky P, et al. : Teniposide and etoposide in previously untreated small-cell lung cancer: a randomized study. Journal of Clinical Oncology 9(9): 1627-1631 1991.

13. Carney ON, Grogan L. Smit EF, et al. : Single-agent oral etoposide for elderly small cell lung cancer patients. Seminars in Oncology 17(1. Suppl 2): 49-53, 1990.

14. Evans WK, Radwi A, Tomiak E, et al. : Oral etoposide and carboplatin: effective therapy for elderly patients with small cell lung cancer. American Journal of Clinical Oncology 18(2): 149-155, 1995.

15. Feld R. Evans WK, DeBoer G, et al. : Combined modality induction therapy without maintenance chemotherapy for small cell carcinoma of the lung. Journal of Clinical Oncology 2(4): 294-304, 1984.

16. Greco FA, Richardson RL, Snell JD et al: Small cell lung cancer: complete remission and improved survival. American Journal of Medicine 66(4): 625-630, 1979.

17. Aisner J, Whitacre M. Van Echo DA, et al. : Combination chemotherapy for small cell carcinoma of the lung: continuous versus alternating non-cross-resistant combinations. Cancer Treatment Reports 66(2): 221-230, 1982.

18. Evans WK. Shepherd FA, Feld R, et al. : VP-16 and cisplatin as first-line therapy for small-cell lung cancer. Journal of Clinical Oncology 3(11):1471-1477, 1985.

19. Skarlos DV, Samantas E, Kosmidis P. et al. : Randomized comparison of etoposide-cisplatin vs. etoposide-carboplatin and irradiation in small-cell lung cancer: a Hellenic Co-operative Oncology Group study. Annals of Oncology 5(7): 601-607 1994.

20. Thatcher N: Ifosfamide/carboplatin/etoposide (ICE) regimen in small cell lung cancer. Lung Cancer 9(Suppl 1): s51-s67, 1993.

21. Cohen MH. Creaven PJ, Fossieck BE, et al. : Intensive chemotherapy of small cell bronchogenic carcinoma. Cancer Treatment Reports 61(3):349-354.   1977,

22. Hansen HH, Dombernowsky P. Hansen M, et al. : Chemotherapy of advanced small-cell anaplastic carcinoma: superiority of a four-drug combination   to a three-drug combination. Annals of Internal Medicine 89(2):177-181,   1978.

23. Jackson DV. Case LD, Zekan PJ, et al. : Improvement of long-term survival   in extensive small-cell lung cancer. Journal of Clinical Oncology 6(7):1161-1169,   1988.

24. Hong WK. Nicaise C, Lawson R, et al. : Etoposide combined with cyclophosphamide plus vincristine compared with doxorubicin plus cyclophosphamide   plus   vincristine   and   with   high-dose cyclophosphamide   plus vincristine in the treatment of small-cell carcinoma of the lung: a randomized trial of the Bristol Lung Cancer Study Group. Journal of Clinical Oncology 7(4): 450-456, 1989,

25. Ettinqer OS: Evaluation of new drugs in untreated patients with small-cell lung cancer: its time has come. ~Journal of Clinical Oncology 8(3): 374-377, 1990.

26. Blackstein M, Eisenhauer EA, Wierzbicki R, et al.: Epirubicin in extensive small-cell lung cancer. A phase II study in previously untreated   patients: a National Cancer Institute of Canada Clinical Trials Group Study. Journal of Clinical Oncology 8(3): 385-389, 1990.

** RECURRENT SMALL-CELL LUNG CANCER **

The prognosis for small-cell carcinoma that has progressed despite chemotherapy is exceedingly poor regardless of stage. Expected median survival is 2-3 months.   Patients who are primarily resistant to chemotherapy and those who have received multiple chemotherapy regimens rarely respond to additional treatment. However, patients who have relapsed more than 6 months following initial treatment are more likely to respond to additional chemotherapy. [1-6]

Some patients with intrinsic endobronchial obstructing lesions or extrinsic compression due to tumor have achieved successful palliation with endobronchial laser therapy, (for endobronchial lesions only) and/or brachytherapy. [7] Patients with progressive intrathoracic tumor after failing initial chemotherapy can achieve significant tumor responses, palliation of symptoms, and short-term local control with external-beam radiotherapy. [8] However, only the rare patient will experience long-term survival following "salvage" radiotherapy. [8]

Patients with central nervous system recurrences can often obtain palliation of symptoms with radiotherapy and/or additional chemotherapy. The majority patients treated with radiotherapy obtain objective responses and improvement following radiotherapy.[9] A retrospective review showed that 43% of patients treated with additional chemotherapy at the time of CNS relapse respond to second-line chemotherapy. [10]

Treatment options:

Palliative radiotherapy. [8]

Salvage chemotherapy. [2-6]

Endobronchial laser therapy and/or brachytherapy. [7]

Clinical trials of phase I or phase II drugs. Refer to the PD0 protocol directory for active clinical trials for patients with small-cell lung cancer.

References:

1. Greco FA: Treatment options for patients with relapsed small cell lung cancer. Lung Cancer 9(Suppl 1): s85-s89, 1993.

2. Johnson OH, Greco FA, Strupp J, et al.: Prolonged administration of oral etoposide in patients with relapsed or refractory small-cell lung cancer: a phase II trial. Journal of Clinical Oncology 8(10):

3. Spiro SG, Souhami RL Geddes ON. et al. : Duration of chemotherapy in small cell lung cancer: a Cancer Research Campaign trial. British Journal of Cancer 59(4)'~ 578-583. 1989.

4. Evans UK. Osoba 0. Feld R, et al. : Etc.poside (VP-16) and cisplatin: an effective treatment for relapse in small-cell lung cancer. Journal of Clinical Oncology 3(1): 65-71. 1985.

5. Gridel C. Contegiacomo A. Lauria R, et al. : Salvage chemotherapy with CCNU and methotrexate for small cell lung cancer resistant to CAV/PE al alternating chemotherapy. Tumor 77(6): 506-510, 1991.

6. Domine M. Lobo F, Jerves N. et al. : Long term survival with salvage chemotherapy in patients with small cell lung cancer (SCLC). Proceedings of the American Society of Clinical Oncology 9: A-938. 242,1990.

7. Miller, JI. Phillips, TW: Neodymium: YAG laser and brachytherapy in the management of inoperable bronchogenic carcinoma. Annals of Thoracic surgery. 50(2): 190-196, 1990.

8. Ochs, JJ. Tester WJ. Cohen MH. et al : Salvage" radiation therapy for intrathoracic small cell carcinoma of the lung progressing on combination chemotherapy. Cancer Treatment Reports 67(12): 1123-1126. 1983

9. Carmichael J. Crane JM, Bunn PA. et al. : Results of therapeutic cranial irradiation in small cell lung cancer. International Journal of Radiation Oncology. Biology. Physics 14(3): 455-459, 1988.

10. Kristensen CA. Kristjansen, PE, Hansen HH: Systemic chemotherapy of brain metastases from small-cell lung cancer: a review Journal of Clinical Oncology 10(9):1498-1502, 1992.

****

This information from POQ is reviewed regularly by members of the P0Q Editorial Boards. If you have specific comments on the content of this information direct them to:

PDQ Editorial Board. ICIC/NCI. 9030 Old Georgetown Rd Bethesda, MD 20892-2650. fax: 301-480-8105. Comments will be forwarded to the Editorial Board for review.

The P00 database also contains listings of clinical trial protocols and directories of organizations and physicians who treat cancer patients, but this information is not available through CancerFax. For more information on accessing PDQ, consult the CancerFax Contents List.

****

(Current as of: 04/01/97)

CHAPTER TWENTY-FOUR

Hospice and the Service It Provides

A service is now available which provides assistance for not only the cancer patient but also some relief to the family. It has been given the name Hospice but such service can be provided by more than one organization in a specific area, all of whom have been certified as a Hospice.

This service becomes available usually when the patient reaches a point where the medical conclusion is that the terminal stage has been reached and death is certain. The timing and recommendation regarding the use of Hospice, at least in my experience, seems to lie with the doctor.

In any major metropolitan area, one is apt find several Hospice services. Some may be managed by local government, others by health organizations and some by hospitals.

All assume the responsibility for the care of the patient including providing a facility to which the patient can be moved. Since this usually takes place at the terminal stage, it can provide a great relief to the family and in particular, the person who has assumed the responsibility of being the primary caretaker.

The following information was derived from our experiences with Hospices in the area in which we live. The name is not revealed as have all identities with respect to those persons and/or agencies who provided various services and assistance for my wife.

As already mentioned, in many metropolitan areas, one is apt to find more than one Hospice. They provide for patients who been classified as terminal and their services are available from the point at which attending physicians decide the patient has become terminal. Normally, this is near the time a person with small cell lung cancer reaches stage 4.

In 1983, legislation was passed by Congress making hospice care a benefit under the Medicare Hospital Insurance Program (Part A). This legislation became effective on November 1, 1982. The bill defines hospice as a public or private organization which primarily operates to provide care to terminally ill individuals and meets the conditions of participation for hospices.

In order to be eligible for hospice under Medicare benefits, the person must be entitled to Part A under Medicare and be certified as being terminally ill. The patient is determined to have a medical life expectancy of six months or less.

Medicare then pays the cost of hospice care in the same manner that it pays for hospitalization.

Many states have made hospice care a benefit under Medicaid. This provides for those who have exhausted their resources and the person's income is not sufficient to pay for all assisted living and medical expenses.

An individual, either directly or through family/caretaker, elects or chooses to accept hospice services through Medicare or Medicaid, whichever applies. During the elected period, only the hospice is entitled to receive Medicare or Medicaid payments. At the same time, the hospice becomes responsible for providing all covered Medicare or Medicaid services relating to the treatment of the terminal condition.

The hospice provides the needed services either through its own resources or through outside providers. The hospice pays the outside providers and is then reimbursed by Medicare of Medicaid. The cost of the patient's care becomes the financial responsibility of the hospice. Whatever the treatment required by the patient, the hospice is totally responsible, both to provide the needs and to pay for them.

It is important to note that hospices enlist the aid of many volunteers. These are people who want to help and they provide tremendous relief to the families of those who are stricken.

A word of thanks does not express sufficient appreciation for what the volunteers are willing to do to help. They represent the spirit of America.

Obtaining the services of a hospice is relatively simple. A telephone call is usually sufficient to set up an appointment to discuss your particular situation. One or more representatives from the hospice will come to your home or another location you may designate. The details will be discussed to include medical treatment, facilities, financial conditions as well as other pertinent topics. You will find that your questions are answered and that there is a desire that you understand completely what signing for hospice care will entail.

If you want to know more about a hospice in your locality, call them. Also, you will find much about hospices on the Internet.

But before you decide on your own to contact a hospice, talk with the attending physician.

* * *

CHAPTER TWENTY-FIVE

RESULTS OF BLOOD TESTS AND THE METAPORT

The following pages contain actual blood tests as well as a picture of the Metaport which had been surgically implanted in Meryl's chest.

Only a few of the multitude of blood tests are included. They were chosen to show the wide range of blood results resulting from her normal levels to those which developed after radiation and chemotherapy.

The number of various tests including bronchoscopys, MRI's, cat scans, etc., plus x-rays too numerous to mention are not included as to the date of the writing of this book, even the records which we provided from previous medical services have not been returned.

The oncologist who treated my wife agreed to let me review his records but it turned out that this was contrary to hospital procedures. I was told that I would have to make a formal request but the copies which they would provide would be at a rather prohibitive charge.

However, my feeling is that there is little more that needs to be included other than a reproduction of the chest x-ray showing the actual tumor in her right lung.

The MRI (Magnetic Resolution Image) which shows the growth pressing on her lower spinal cord was not visible on the x-rays. A reproduction of this result also might be of interest but this too has not been made available to me.

The colossal amount of records, papers, x-rays, etc., has left me with a great deal of wonderment as to whether or not all this was necessary. After all, from the beginning, it was known what the outcome would be. Was there and is there really any need to add more misery to the few weeks that she had with the almost robotic way these tests were constantly done. Regardless of what the tests showed, she would have been subjected to the same treatment. Keeping her up most of the night in order to take these tests is certainly not in keeping with "First, do no harm."

If I have learned anything at all from what I have seen and experienced, it would be that if it is true that conventional treatment adds a few days to one's life, then the quality of the remaining days of life does not fit into the equation. Certainly, what time is left is not time that one can enjoy. The treatment causes such agony and pain that precious few days are such that the patient feels up to any feeling of appreciation for being alive.

Yes, the will to live is one of the strongest we experience but in time, the destruction of our mental and physical processes also removes the desire to continue living.

Having gone through this experience, I can understand why a person might want to put an end to all the suffering. While I personally don't agree with Euthanasia as it conflicts with my religious and personal beliefs, it is only the person who is experiencing the debilitation of life's processes who must make this decision. Yet, throughout the greatest of suffering, it has always been my thought that perhaps at the last minute, someone would find a cure for the affliction. Should this happen and life had been ended prematurely, the cure could have never been applied.

* * *

DATE: March 12 1996
PATIENT : Meril Abraham
PHYSICIAN: Dr. Jaime Narvaez

TEST	RESULT	REFERENCE RANGE	UNITS
CBC/DIFFERENTIAL:			
HGB	15.4	12.0—16.0	g/dl
HCT	45	39 — 47	%
MCHC	34	30-34	%
WBC	7150	5000 — 10000	cels/oc
RBC	5.0	4.0 — 5.5.	M/uL
PLATELET COUNT	315	150 450	K/iA
DEFFERENTIAL:			
Lymphocytes	32	13 - 45	%
Monocytes	4	3-10	%
Eosinophils	2	1 - 4	%
Basophils	0	0 - 1	%
Neutrophils	62	50 - 70	%
Stab.	0	2—7	%
Remarks:			

Note: The blood reports given by this clinic cover 3 pages. For the purposes of this book, only the page showing the blood counts is reproduced.

* * *

NAME: ABRAHAM   MERYL
ACN :   10281735
AGE :   71 YRS   SEX: F   ROOM *:
COLLECTION DATE   04/25/96   08:20

TEST	RESULT	RANGE	UNITS	TEST	R ESULT	RANGE	UNITS

Profiles

CHEM 24 PROFILE

TEST	RESULT	RANGE	UNITS	TEST	RESULT	RANGE	UNITS
GLUCOSE	119 HI	70-105	mg/dl	GLOBULIN	2.7	2.3—3.5	gm/dl
BUN	12	0.7-18	mg/dl	A/G RATIO	1.4	1.0—2.3	gm/dl
CREATININE	0.8	0.7—1.3	mg/dl	TOTAL BILl	0..5	0.4—1.4	mg/dl
SODIUM	139	135—145	mEq/L	DIRECT BILl	0.10	0.00—0.26	mg/dl
POTASSIUM	3.4 LO	3.5—5.0	mEqfL	ALK PHOS	152 HI	0—145	U/L
CHLORIDE	101	98—109	mEq/L	GGT	78 HI	0—70	U/L
C02	25	22—33	mEq/L	SGOT (AST)	40	0—52	U/L
ELECT.BAL	16	4—18	mEq/L	SGPT (ALT)	48	0—52	U/L
URIC ACID	2.7	2.6—6.0	mg/dl	LDH	217	50—260	U/L
PHOSPHORUS	3.1	2.5—5.0	mg/dl	CPK	43	41—117	U/L
CALCIUM	8.4	8.4—10.2	mg/dl	TRIG	43	35—135	mg/dl
T. PROTEIN	6.6	6.0—8.3	gm/dl	CHOLESTEROL	227 HI	0—200	mg/dl
ALBUMIN	3.9	3.2—5.5	gm/dl				

            < 200 MG/DL — DESIRABLE
              200—239 MG/DL — BORDERLINE
            > 240 MG/DL — HIGH RISK

COMPLETE BLOOD COUNT

TEST	RESULT	RANGE	UNITS	TEST	RESULT	RANGE	UNITS
PLATELETS	588 HI	130—400	x10'3	MCV	95.1	80—100	um~3
WBC	4.9	4.8—10.8	xlO'3	MCH	32.1	26—34	pg
R8C	3.18 LO	4.0—5.5	x10~6	MCHC	33.7	31.0—37.0	gm/dl
HEMOGLOBIN	10.2 LO	12—16	gm/dl	ROW	12.9	11.5—14.5	%
HEMATOCRIT	30.2 LO	36—46	%				

DIFFERENTIAL

TEST	RESULT	RANGE	UNITS	TEST	RESULT	RANGE	UNITS
NEUTROPHIL	68.3	40—74	%	LYMPHOCYTE	28.3	19—48	%
MONOCYTE	3.4	3.4—9.0	%				

                 * * *

NAME: ABRAHAM   MERYL
ACN   10307667
AGE   :   71 YRS   SEX: F

COLLECTION DATE   :   05/28/96

TEST	RESULT	RANGE	UNITS	TEST	RESULT	RANGE	UNITS

Profiles

CHEM 24 PROFILE

TEST	RESULT		RANGE	UNITS	TEST	RESULT		RANGE	UNITS
GLUCOSE	94		70—105	mg/dl	GLOBULIN	2.1	LO	2.3—3.5	gm/dl
BUN	15		7—18	mg/dl	A/G RATIO	1.8		1.0—2.3	gm/dl
CREATININE	0.9		0.7—1.3	mg/dl	TOTAL BIL1	0.3	LO	0.4—1.4	mg/dl
SODIUM	137		135—145	mEq/L	DIRECT BIL1	0.00		0.00—0.26	mg/dl
POTASSIUM	5.3	HI	3.5—5.0	mEq/L	ALK PHOS	162	HI	0—145	U/L
CHLORIDE	102		98—109	mEq/L	GGT	50		0—70	U/L
CO2	21	LO	22—33	mEq/L	SGOT (AST)	18		0—52	U/L
ELECT.BAL.	19	HI	4—18		SGPT (ALT)	35		0—52	U/L
URIC ACID	2.4	LO	2.6—6.0	mg/dl	LDH	311	HI	50—260	U/L
PHOSPHORUS	3.5		2.5—5.0	mg/dl	CPK	20	LO	41—117	U/L
CALCIUM	8.3	LO	8.4—10.2	mg/dl	TRIG	171	HI	35—135	mg/dl
T. PROTEIN	5.8	LO	6.0—8.3	gm/dl	CHOLESTEROL	143		0—200	mg/dl
Albumin	3.7		3.2—5.5	gm/dl					

```
                                  < 200 MG/DL - DESIRABLE
                                  200—239 MG/DL - BORDERLINE
                                > 240 MG/DL - HIGH RISK
```

HEPATIC PROFILE

TEST	RESULT		RANGE	UNITS
IRON	260	HI	50—200	ug/dl

COMPLETE BLOOD COUNT

TEST	RESULT		RANGE	UNITS	TEST	RESULT		RANGE	UNITS
PLATELETS	134		130—400	x10~3	MCV	91.8		80—100	um~3
WBC	42.9	HI	4.8—10.8	x10"3	MCH	31.6		26—34	pg
RBC	3.07	LO	4.0—5.5	x10~6	MCHC	34.4		31.0—37.0	gm/dl
HEMOGLOBIN	9.7	LO	12—16	gm/dl	RDW	19.7	HI	11.5—14.5	%
HEMATOCRIT	28.2	LO	36—46	%					

DIFFERENTIAL

TEST	RESULT		RANGE	UNITS	TEST	RESULT		RANGE	UNITS
NEUTROPHIL	84.0	HI	40—74	%	LYMPHOCYTE	10.0	LO	19—48	%
MONOCYTE	2.0	LO	3.4—9.0	%					

                              * * *

MRN: 296180940 Name: ABRAHAM   MERYL   R.   LABORATORY

*** Labs Daily for 21-MAY-1996 11:33:25.40 to 20-MAY-1996 11:33:25.40 ***

POTASSIUM	COL: 05/21/96 10:00 STAT		ACC# T62867
POTASSIUM	*3.2	mmol/L	[3.7-5.3]

METABOLIC PANEL	COL: 05/21/96 06:57 ROUTINE		ACC# T62422
CALCIUM	*3.6	MEQ/L	[4.3-5.2]
INORG PHOSPHATE	*2.3	MG/DL	[2.5-4.5]
MAGNESIUM	*1.9	MEQ/L	[1.4-1.8]
URIC ACID	*1.1	MG/DL	[2.5-6.8]
GLUCOSE	*139	MG/DL	[65-115]
SODIUM	*132	mmol/L	[136-146]
POTASSIUM	*3.6	mmol/L	[3.7-5.3]
CHLORIDE	*109	mmol/L	[96-106]
CARBON DIOXIDE	*20	mmol/L	[21-31]
TOTAL PROTEIN	*4.1	GM/DL	[6.1-8.2]
ALBUMIN	*2.2	GM/DL	[3.8-5.1]
BUN	10	MG/DL	[5-24]
CREATININE	*0.6	MG/DL	[0.7-1.3]

DIFF-ELECTRONIC	COL: 05/21/9606:57 ROUTINE		ACC# T62422
GRANS ELECTRONIC	*22.0	%	[50-70]
LYMPHS ELECTRONIC	*66.2	%	[25-401
MONOCYTE ELECTRONIC	7.6	%	
LYMPHOCYTES ABSOLUTE	*0.8	K/ul	[1.5-4.0]
MONO ABSOLUTE	0.1	K/ul	[0.1-0.8]
GRANULOCYTES ABSOLUTE			
	*0.3	K/ul	[1.5-7.0]
BASO ELECTRONIC	0.4	%	
EOS ELECTRONIC	3.8	%	
EOS ABSOLUTE	0.0	K/ul	
BASO ABSOLUTE	0.0	K/ul	
PLATELET COMMENT	PLATELETS DECREASED		
RBC COMMENTS	ANISOCYTOSIS		
	1+		
	HYPOCHROMIC		
	2+		

CBC	COL: 05/21/96 06:57 ROUTINE		ACC# T62422
WBC COUNT	*12	K/uL	[5-10]
RBC COUNT	*2.35	M/uL	[4.2-5.4]
HEMOGLOBIN	*7.8	G/DL	[12.0-16.0]

HEMATOCRIT	*22. 8	%	[37-47]
MEAN CELL VOLUME	97.2	fL	[82-99]
MEAN CELL HGB CONC	34.1	G/dL	[32-36]
RBC DISTRIBUTION	*15.4		[11.5-14.5]
PLATELET COUNT	*20	K/uL	[150-400]
MEAN PLATELET VOLUME	8.1	FL	[6.2-10.6]

DIFFERENTIAL MANUAL

BAND NEUTROPHIL	5	%	[0-7]

* * *

184

The top end of the tubing was inserted into the large vein which is located near the neck and under the shoulder bone.

The device at the bottom of the picture is the actual twin port. It is implanted into the chest and the needle is inserted into either of the two ports. The area under the two circles and at the entrance to the ports were the places where the clots would occur.

This is a picture of the actual Metaport which was implanted in Meryl's chest.

DAILY RECORDS I

I began keeping daily memos during my wife's illness beginning with our return from Juarez, Mexico, until she died. The closeness that developed between us as her cancer progressed was an important factor in deciding on a written record.

The entries included a great deal of everyday events in order to better portray the magnitude of accepting full responsibility for my wife's care and well being.

We all go about our daily lives with little thought to what conditions would be like if some major catastrophe were to occur. When that crisis comes, it usually is sudden and unexpected. If plans had not been made prior to the event, it may be too late to do so after the fact.

Life must continue in all aspects to the extent possible as everyday responsibilities must be given time or else one must find people who will perform these tasks. I was not successful in finding anyone to bring in on a daily or even part-time basis who was satisfactory to my wife. She has always been a very particular person and our experience with outside help has not always been acceptable to her satisfaction, except in a few instances.

It never occurred to me to hire someone on my own volition who would not please Meryl. While there are many people who would have been eminently satisfactory, the overwhelming daily demand on time left little opportunity for interviews. The few people with whom I did talk were not acceptable.

There were other personal considerations for her, such as all her hair falling out and the loss of weight. She needed constant attention and I'm not sure she was willing for me to assign that responsibility to a stranger. Perhaps a better way to put this would be that because she went through so much pain, nausea and suffering, she was not willing to allow others to see her in this condition.

Finally, my wife told me repeatedly that she felt that my attending her was what was keeping her alive. She mentioned this to others. I suppose that my own apprehension of a further deterioration in her spirits and morale, as well as an increase in the fear she already had, added to my unwillingness to change.

Those who might find themselves in this unfortunate position may benefit from this daily record. That is my purpose in providing them as a part of this book.

* * *

BEGINNING WITH RETURN FROM JUAREZ, MEXICO

March 19, 1996

Returned today from Juarez, Mexico, about 5 p.m. Left warm weather at 6:30 p.m., with temperatures in the 80's. Long trip with three stops. Weather a little rough with very bumpy landings. Was so tired when I went to bed that I don't remember anything after that.

Going to hospital tomorrow where Meryl will enter to see what situation is now. My mind is now adjusted to whatever will happen. Was raining when got back but snowed during night. Tomorrow is the first day of spring.

Got to a point in Mexico where I could converse a little in Spanish. I think that with a little more time there as well as time to study a little, could become fairly proficient in the language. Wrote a letter in French for one of the nurses who has a French boyfriend. That was an interesting exercise changing Spanish to French but we got it done.

It was four weeks ago that we left. Michele picked us up at airport and Dan was waiting at house. Susan brought boys over and prepared dinner. It was a nice homecoming.

I intend to keep a daily log from now on to the extent possible. Since I did not keep a log while in Mexico, I am going to reconstruct the events that occurred there from memory. These are included in this first entry which I hope to keep on a daily basis. It is my belief that a daily record may prove valuable at some time in the future as conventional treatment of my wife's disease begins.

Meryl began to experience pains in her back late in 1995 after she had been in a dentist's chair for about four hours while he removed some upper teeth and replaced them with implants. She went to see a

187

chiropractor who had been recommended to her by one of her best friends and she had been seeing for some time.

He worked on her back for over an hour without success. Then when he discovered a partial denture in her mouth, he told her the problem was the dental work that had been done. She felt he had accomplished some improvements.

As the days went by, her back pain began to diminish but she began to experience pain in her right leg. Again, she made an appointment with the chiropractor, but this time she was unable to obtain relief.

As Christmas, 1995 approached, Michele took her to a clinic nearby where she received special massages on her back and legs. These seem to help but it was evident on Christmas day at our annual family gift opening that she was not feeling well. At that time, none of us realized the severity of the pain she was experiencing. Looking back, this is one of the circumstances for which all of us had regrets. I could not help feeling that perhaps I was not sufficiently concerned.

Finally, in January, Dan convinced her to see his doctor. He made an appointment for Meryl about the middle of January with a doctor who had been giving him annual physicals. He began a number of tests focused on her back and leg pain. Finally in February, she was scheduled for an MRI, (Magnetic Resolution Image), a chest x-ray and a mammogram. A consultation was scheduled with the family and the doctor announced that the mammogram showed that her breasts were clear. I breathed easier at that point. This made the next announcement all the more difficult to accept.

With hardly a breath in between, the doctor's next words were, "But there is nothing we can do with the lung cancer".

The shock from that statement is one from which I have yet to recover. He stated further that no surgery was indicated and that he needed to schedule her for a biopsy to determine what type of cancer she had.

All this was on Monday morning, February 19. The shock we all experienced was totally numbing. It was more than I could handle so abruptly. On the way back from the doctor's office, I was unable to keep my mind on my driving.

After arriving home, my lack of control resulted in tears on my part. I became embarrassed that at a time when she needed reinforcement and strength from me, I was the one who became weak. I apologized and assured her that this would not happen again. However, my breaking down seemed to give her some strength, just when she needed it most. I think that for a brief moment, her concern for me overcame her own fear of the cancer.

Meryl contacted her very close friend whom she had known about five years and had a predisposition against conventional treatment. The woman and her husband began to investigate places where alternative treatment was available. The friend called back and said they had located a clinic in Juarez, Mexico, which also had an office in El Paso, Texas. She was to talk with the doctor the following morning to make arrangements to go there.

After another conversation, my wife told me that they wanted to fly the two of us to El Paso in their private plane and wanted to leave immediately. They had planned the trip to take place in two days with an overnight stop in Oklahoma. The notice was short but the urgency was great. Meryl was completely opposed to radiation and chemotherapy.

Friends of ours had gone through this in previous years and we had seen what conventional treatment had done to them before they died. A surgeon who was a good friend of ours had told us years before that chemotherapy was nothing more than a poison which in most cases, was nothing more than a death warrant.

We were not able to leave the next day but the plan now was to leave on Wednesday, February 21, sometime in the morning. Weather and other matters forced a delay, but we finally departed early in the afternoon.

The first part of the flight was fairly smooth but we did encounter some rain. We had to change our flight plan because of the late departure and the fact we stopped short of our planned destination for that day. I was relieved as it was about 9 p.m. when we landed and after 10 p.m. when we finally found transportation to take us to a motel.

After we checked in and were settled, our friends came over to see Meryl. At that point, she was in a great deal of pain, broke down completely and cried for some time. We tried to console her and finally, after we were alone, she was able to go to sleep.

Thursday morning found her in better spirits. She asked me to go to a store for some supplies we would need in Juarez. From there, we went to the airport and a short time later, started what was to be the second and final leg of our journey. I was very stressed because I knew she had been in pain the day before.

As we continued our flight, the weather deteriorated with high head winds. The turbulence caused her pain to increase and I was suffering with her. Fortunately, she had asked me to get some seasickness medicine before we left Columbus. At least, she did not experience nausea along with leg pains.

The turbulence got worse and our air speed dropped to a point where we were making little progress. We finally landed early in the afternoon for fuel. While on the ground, the wind continued to increase and it was decided to stay over in Lubbeck, Texas, hoping that the wind would die down by morning.

I noticed that Meryl was having a little difficulty walking, but did not complain. We checked into a motel and had lunch. By that time, it was late in the afternoon and we spent the rest of the day in our rooms. That night, Meryl once more became very fearful and agitated, and we needed to calm her.

Friday morning, the weather looked better and it seemed that the wind had died down somewhat. However, the closer we came to El Paso, the worse the head winds became. At times, our air speed dropped to as low as fifty-five knots or about fifty eight to sixty miles per hour. The turbulence at times was terrible, and I was frustrated at not being able to provide any comfort to the pain my wife was experiencing.

We landed in El Paso an hour late but the driver was still waiting for us. He took us to their El Paso office, to Juarez so we could check into our motel, and then immediately to the clinic.

After an initial examination, we returned to our motel and the four of us went out to dinner. Meryl had very little appetite, did not eat much of what she ordered. This would be the last time during our stay that she would eat anywhere except in the motel room or the clinic.

Treatment started the next day and the doctor provided a great deal of encouragement, including his belief that tests made were not indicative of cancer. We had been told not to have a biopsy done at home and had canceled the one scheduled in Columbus, as this was to be done at the clinic.

The doctor went through the lab results item by item. He said everything was in the normal range, and the kidneys and liver were in excellent condition.

We were to be in Juarez until March 19. During this time, she was given chelation to clear her body of impurities and heavy metals; colonics to help clear her colon; and a variety of medication, including shark cartilage, to strengthen her immune system. I did not realize until after our return home that she had also been given live cell injection and was treated orally with Laetrile.

To summarize the stay in Mexico, the significant point was that the pain in her legs worsened and became unbearable at times. Also, because her veins were being punctured too many times, the staff put in a temporary port in her upper right chest where all fluids were inserted. This was done surgically and resulted in a partial collapse of her right lung.

We called the doctor, who came to the motel and decided she should stay in the clinic that night. He drove both of us there. The surgeon, who was called, said after examining her that the collapse was not serious and she would recover shortly.

The leg pains reached a point where at times they were unbearable. Walking became more and more difficult. Occasionally the pain was so intense we had to ask the doctor to see her in the motel. It was a source of relief that he was always willing to come to her, no matter when we called him.

By the time we were ready to leave Juarez, and we were delayed a couple of days because we both wanted to talk with doctors in two other clinics there, walking for her had become almost impossible. From the time we arrived at the airport in El Paso for our return trip and until after treatment began at home, we had to utilize a wheelchair. Walking just a couple of steps was excruciating for her.

When we arrived in Columbus, I was pushing her in her wheelchair while carrying three bags over my shoulders when our daughter Michele met us. We picked up our checked luggage and returned home. It was good to be back, and I think Meryl found joy in being home also. The fact our family was waiting and showed such great concern was the best of morale builders.

The appointment for the next day for a cancer examination was temporarily forgotten in the pleasure of reunion.

March 20, 1996

Got to hospital and news was not good. Test that doctor wanted to do to find out what kind of cancer my wife had was not done because of her emotional reaction to information about her condition. Several tests are now rescheduled for Friday.

Had visitors tonight until after 11 p.m. Am so far behind on so many urgent items, checks to write, taxes, etc., but no time. This is the first day of spring but it snowed most of night as well as all day. Snow on ground is now about five inches deep. Unless it really warms up tomorrow, I will have to get on tractor to clear snow. Meantime, have two empty apartments with people waiting to occupy them, but cannot get to them for time being to put in rentable condition. Times have become tedious but again, will attempt to face the opportunities head on.

I am not getting much done. News at hospital has started a whole new emotional reaction. I'm okay and am holding up very well. Situation is very demanding and it is a twenty-four-hour daily situation. Real problem is her emotional state, which is terribly negative. It's something I have feared for many years and the reaction unfortunately is exactly as I have anticipated. Concern for Meryl is my top priority.

March 22, 1996

Weather has been nice here for the last couple of days. Really windy yesterday and a huge tree came down, torn out at the roots by an apparent gust of wind. Just missed tearing up neighbors' patio. Tree must be over 100 feet long so big job ahead of cutting it up. May try to contact a timber cutter as there ought to be some really good lumber in the tree.

Have a daily routine of taking Meryl for radiation treatments. New X-rays, Cat scan of brain as well as other tests now complete. Brain scan came out okay as did mammogram. Problem seems to be in right lung and spine.

Pain has become a major problem because of restriction in lower lumbars around spinal cord. Left leg in particular has terrible pain. Haven't been able to do much of anything as demand on time has been almost around the clock. Radiation therapy is scheduled everyday, five days a week. Also tomorrow, a bone scan is scheduled.

Am trying to get taxes done but not much luck. Perhaps schedule will settle down after radiation has a chance to have an effect. She is using a heating pad on back and legs constantly except when she is up or at hospital. At night, I am applying an ointment to both her legs, with hot wet towels afterward for about fifteen minutes. As soon as possible, I will purchase more heating pads so that I can keep her legs warm. That seems to reduce the pain.

March 28, 1996

Another long day with more bad news. Spent good part of day at hospital with third radiation treatment on spine and bone scan. Think that amount of radiation, including injection for bone scan, was too much for her. Got home about 3 p.m. Michele was here, and I went out to get new pain prescriptions. Someone had to be with her at all times. I had to go to another druggist that carried the prescribed drugs. Finally returned about 5 p.m.. Dan stopped by with boys for about two hours, then left for home. Tomorrow, will go for another radiation treatment at 11:15 a.m., then to lab for blood work. At clinic in Juarez, blood work was done every week. Here, not one has been done so far. Had to bring it up this morning, so they agreed to scheduling for tomorrow. Another radiation treatment tomorrow, then a consultation with oncologist at 12:30. They want to start chemotherapy as well as radiation. Will have to wait to see what happens.

Meryl is not happy with the idea of conventional treatment.

I am holding up fairly well except that am rather tired by evening. There is no break from morning to night but if this effort provides help in her quality of life, that will give me great gratification. Still cold with a little rain with more scheduled for tomorrow. But Sunday will be in 60's and sunny. Busy day at hospital today with family conference with lead physician.

The biopsy has determined that Meryl has small cell lung cancer. This is the worst kind of news with a lot of emotion. Dan and Michele were both there, as well as a close family friend. After radiation treatment tomorrow morning, have appointment with oncologist to determine extent of chemotherapy. Dan was to fly to Chicago. He put it off to be at consultation. Was able to get on a standby status for flight tonight at 9 p.m. Apparently made it okay, as we haven't heard from him. It's about 10:30 and as usual am tired. Have had some weird experiences with meditation.

March 29, 1996

Left for medical facility about 10:30 a.m. and finally got home after 6 p.m. After the radiation treatment, had appointment with oncologist as I've mentioned. He wanted to start chemo today with an IV. Said it would take about an hour, but it was more like four hours. Now, she takes the chemo orally for the next four days. Then, nothing except radiation treatments for next three weeks. Then, another round of chemo.

Doctor told her that if she stayed on pain pills alone, he would give her just three weeks to live.

Tumor on lung is about the size of an egg. The type is small cell and has spread to spine. That is what is causing discomfort as lesion is pressing against spinal chord causing pain in back and legs. However, brain, liver, bladder, kidneys and other organs are all okay.

She is also taking supplements from her stay at clinic in Juarez which I think will help counter the side effects of the chemo. Am a bit tired as usual but much is a result of my concern for my wife.

March 30, 1977

My throat is a little sore, with slight temperature. Worse problems are possibility of passing this on to Meryl and getting to hospital every day for radiation treatments. Now she is on pills to be taken for four days. Then chemo stops for I believe about three weeks but radiation treatment to back continues, five days a week. None on Saturday or Sunday because clinic is closed but it starts again on Monday. Appointment with oncologist on Tuesday afternoon which is also the last day of pills for this session. My sense is that tumor in lung is inoperable. Am going to Vicks myself up tonight. Want to go to church tomorrow as it is Palm Sunday and I usually pick up new palm. With her immune system dropping as a result of chemo, don't want to add to current problem by passing on germs. Had planned to finish cutting top of fallen tree tomorrow, but rain is predicted. Will only be able to cut down to main trunk which must be at least two feet in diameter, and it may be over fifty-feet long. So, will have to get someone in to cut it up as my chain saw is too small for the size of tree.

March 31, 1996

Piled the Vicks on last night as well as taking 2,000 mg of vitamin C, the Echinacea herb, and a few other medications. Woke up wet from perspiration about 4 a.m. but didn't dare to get out of bed and risk a chill. Finally got up about 6:50, cleaned up and dressed, light breakfast and then to Mass at 8 a.m.

Left Mass just a little early as I didn't want to be away too long. While not quite well, am much better than last night.

Michele is here. Meryl is having the worst day yet. Looks as though she will not get out of bed for the first time since all this started. When we see the oncologist Tuesday, will ask him about lung surgery. My belief is that it may be too late. Am concerned about pain and lack of appetite. She is down 30 pounds in such a very short time. Pain is draining energy and causing nausea.

I still have a sinus infection but perhaps this time, will try mind over matter for a change.

April 1 , 1996

Phone went out of order yesterday and it is still out today. Had a combination of rain and sleet. An hour and a half later, we had an accumulation of about two inches of real wet snow. Had to clear off the station wagon and clear a path on driveway prior to leaving for radiation treatment. Not only was it cold but very windy. So much in fact that wind was causing a buzzing sound that was sort of startling. I seem to be keeping a sort of status quo with my sinus infection or cold, whichever it is. The good news is that it is supposed to warm up this afternoon with sunshine.

Called telephone company from a neighbor's house and they promised to get somebody out right away. Explained the urgency. Radiation treatment tomorrow morning. Then appointment with oncologist. She takes the last of chemo pills tomorrow morning for this cycle of treatment. Michele left for Amarillo, Texas, then San Antonio and finally Salt Lake City. Will be back on Friday. Dan got back from Chicago last night. Good news is that snow has all melted, sun is out and warming up but wind is fierce. Also, phone is back on and sound is very clear.

Am sort of wishing phone was still out. Seems like it has been ringing ever since I found dial tone was back. Don't know what they did but ring is louder, volume is higher and sound is crystal clear.

Came up to shave this morning and just as I entered the upstairs bedroom door, my right leg practically gave way with me. Had the most violent pain from the knee down to my ankle. Came on suddenly, lasted about five minutes and left just as suddenly. Am now thinking it was some kind of a cramp. Also checked to make sure that I'm not pregnant and found that was not the case. Anyway, feel pretty good tonight but nose is a little drippy. But believe that am getting away with an easy bout this time.

April 2, 1996

Long day again. Left this morning for medical facility with the idea that we would be back by 2 p.m. or so. Not so. Radiation machines were down and we had to wait almost an hour before getting treatment. That got us to doctor appointment about 12:40. With acute nausea, it was impossible to give her the last of her chemo capsules. Today was to be the last for this cycle. Doctor decided that several problems could be solved by giving last treatment via IV. So, didn't get home until after 6 p.m., but nausea was gone and she was feeling much better. Even ate, but not too much. Still, more than last several days. The first round of chemo is now over with a four-week layoff before the next round begins. Not sure how many more radiation treatments are planned. The new round of prescriptions today cost almost $2,000. I thought the one last Friday was expensive at almost $500 but today's came as a total surprise. Luckily, insurance covers a great deal of it. Total bills to date must be well over $30,000. I know that I've written checks for almost $15,000. Problem is that neither Medicare nor Aetna will pay for treatment in Juarez. Had to miss Internal Revenue Service work again, and only three more sessions left. Michele called from San Antonio tonight. She changed her reservation from the airport motel to the Holiday on the river at my suggestion. Was thrilled at location and sights. She had never been to San Antonio before. I was surprised as I thought that she has been in practically every major city in the USA.

April 3, 1996

Beautiful today. Went for radiation treatment and we were in and out in less than 10 minutes. First time for everything. Helper showed up at 1 p.m. so we got a lot more of the tree cut. Saw was acting up and had to quit. Got a broken blister on my finger from just pulling the rope to start saw. Gas may have had water in it. Was rather tired so quit for the day. Will take a warm bath before retiring. Going to oncologist after radiation tomorrow to learn how to do Neupogen injections for the next 10 days. Drug is to build up bone marrow so that white blood counts are brought back to normal. Chemo destroys some bone marrow and interferes with production of red and white cells. Time changes today.

April 4, 1996

Days are up and down. There are fairly good days relatively speaking and bad days. But that's to be expected. Was trained today to give injections. For the next 10 days, I have to give her an injection in the stomach each day of a drug called Neupogen. The ten vials for the 10 days, one per day had a cost of over $1,400. Three other pain and nausea prescriptions added another nearly $400. Told the doctor that if he could anticipate ahead of time and give me the prescriptions a few days in advance, could get them filled at Wright Patterson Air Force Base because of my military service. He promised to do. Still raining outside. If this keeps up, we will be seeing floods.

April 5, 1996

Weather is running about 20 degrees or so below normal. Day went rather well but pain and nausea still persist. However, her appetite is coming back as well as her spirits. Gave her another Neupogen injection today but counts are beginning to drop.

April 6, 1996

Not a good day for wife but, by extra special urging, got her to eat a half grilled cheese sandwich, a little juice and hot chocolate with marshmallows. That is most she has eaten in several days. Just finished setting clocks ahead an hour. Expect to go to Mass tomorrow morning and didn't want to find myself an hour late. Even remembered to reset time on PC. This has been a busy day without a break until now. When sister-in-law left this afternoon, rode with her to wife's office to pick up her car. It had been parked there since early in February. Michele had driven it several times. Have it here now and will use it on trips to hospital as it is more comfortable than station wagon. Almost had a blizzard here in afternoon. About two inches of snow fell in less than forty-five minutes. Ground is still white but snow has melted on walks, roads and drives. Was going to bake a couple of hams today but no time.

April 7, 1966

Tried cutting more tree, but chain saw still acting up. Will take it apart tomorrow and see what is wrong. While Meryl is eating again, she still does not have much appetite. Daily Neupogen shots continue. Medication is now seven times a day as well. As we approach what is called a critical period after chemotherapy treatment, her appetite has been dropping.

April 8, 1996

Went to hospital for radiation treatment and blood work. It was a Monday morning when everyone should have stayed home. Got there and there were no wheelchairs available. Took almost forty minutes to find one, then discovered that wheelchair automatic doors were not working so had to go clear around to another entrance although there were lots of people around but nobody offered to hold a door open. Even though we got to hospital forty minutes early, we ended up being three minutes late for radiation. Then we were told that it would be awhile before they could get to her and to go ahead and get blood work done. Went to that section but girl at reception desk was too busy with personal phone call and blowing her nose to help. Finally, after about eight minutes, she wanted to know if we wanted anything. Told her we were there for blood work but she couldn't find order. So a series of phone calls was made with no success. Then I got on the phone with my patience exhausted and the order came through. Next, we waited another half hour before someone was available to take blood. Went back down to radiation and they were still behind. Had to put spouse on a bed by this time as she was tired and in pain. I felt I had had it, and said to the powers-that-be I thought the day must be considered " be cruel to patients day". That stirred things and all at once, head doctor, administrator, and others, all wanted to talk with me. At the same time, I had let drop that the head of department would hear from me. That seemed to get some attention. The entire day was taken to give my wife whatever support I could. Watching all her constant pain prompted my actions. It is the most stressful thing I have ever been through, but that is nothing compared with what she is suffering. Another Neupogen shot today.

April 9, 1997

Since I had Internal Revenue Service volunteer duty today, arrived at hospital an hour early and what a change. Everyone was bending over backward. The doctor in charge of radiology took over personally. He checked her right away for new pain in hip, had an X-ray taken, personally pushed the wheel chair to the elevator and X-ray section, ordered work to be done, and left instructions to be called as soon as the film was processed. Meryl no sooner came out of X-ray when the doctor and his assistant both came in to check the film. They announced there was no new problem and all was okay. That was good news. Was only a half hour late at IRS office, which was quite busy. This is the last afternoon with one more session Thursday night. Then, April 15 comes on Monday so we're all finished for another year.

So another long day and will be glad to get to bed, but radiation ends Friday and the shots I am giving her end on Saturday.

In the meantime, have gotten behind on taxes. Will have to get an extension on personal income tax but all business returns are done except for about an hour's work. Would have finished but didn't have enough forms.

It's unbelievable the amount of flowers and food coming in. Refrigerator is full and stays that way. The ham that I baked is making a big hit with spouse, Dan, Susan and Michele.

Michele joined us for dinner tonight. I prepared warmed-up buttered ham, baked chunk potatoes and cabbage rolls. Also, lime Jello with crushed pineapple. Meryl ate the whole thing, unusual for her.

* * *

199

DAILY RECORDS II

April 10, 1966

Got to hospital a little early but the radiologist wanted to see spouse. Problem was that after waiting forty five minutes, it got to be too much, so told the nurse that Meryl couldn't take anymore for today. Will see doctor tomorrow. Two more radiation treatments tomorrow and Friday. Also three more Neupogen shots that I have to give, ending on Saturday. Will be happy when wife is able to feel better and develop an appetite.

April 11, 1966

It has been a beautiful day, weather wise. I think the warmest day yet. Left for hospital about 10:25 a.m. Dan came in for awhile. He has an argument to present before the Sixth Circuit court next Monday. One more radiation treatment after today. Blood was also taken. Tomorrow morning, final treatment and conference with radiologist.

Went to post office and then returned to make copies of parts of taxes. All now in the mail, except extension for our personal return. Also, final IRS duty tonight so feel sense of relief. Last shots tomorrow and Saturday. Think that Meryl is getting better but she doesn't believe it. Don't know if all the agony brings any credit to medical profession. To put a patient through all this seems almost inhuman.

April 12, 1996

The combination of vitamin C and Echinacea really made short work of my semi-annual sinus infection. Aside for a couple days of sniffles and the first night of temperature, hardly noticed it. Have been a great believer of the herbal anti-biotic and now, even more so.

Meryl had last radiation treatment today. Conference with doctor not very satisfactory. We were kept waiting for almost a half hour. By the time she had been in the wheel chair for an hour, she had become too ill to do blood work doctor wanted. Forgot to get a prescription renewed but remembered after we arrived home. Spent over three hours on telephone and finally got a nurse who seemed to care. Then had to drive to a special pharmacy to get drug, which contained a narcotic. Didn't get home until after 6 p.m.

Found Meryl in terrible pain so performed special massage and hot towel application, gave her a pain pill and within about fifteen minutes she was comfortable. She even ate a fairly decent supper. Michele stopped by and left about half hour ago. I was going to get a haircut today but had to put it off. The back of my head is actually becoming most uncomfortable. Noticed that spring flowers including forsythia are all in bloom today. Happened overnight.

April 13, 1996

Didn't have to go to hospital today. But had a lot to do. Earlier, some book work, regular routine of pills, supplements, a little breakfast, etc. Then, sister-in-law came over to wash wife's hair. She agreed to stay until I returned some items to library, got a haircut and went to the post office. In the meantime, had taken battery out of wife's car to turn in when I buy a new one. New young barber didn't do a good job on my hair and I had to make him redo part of back and sides. Really looked terrible but after he trimmed it some more, wasn't too bad. It will grow out again. Got back about 1:30, got some lunch and made ready for last shot. Sister-in-law didn't want to see the injection, so she took off just before the needle found its mark. What a relief. Glad it's over for now, at least. Then, went out and purchased new battery as well as a few other items.

When I got back, she was asleep. I installed battery in her car and everything worked fine. She was hungry tonight, so cooked up some thinly sliced potatoes with butter, salt, pepper, parsley leaves and basil. Took about fifteen minutes for them to get done. Meantime, had to go to grocery to get some special mustard she wanted as well as a sweet onion. Out of season but supermarket had some from Brazil. So, cooked some all beef wieners, a couple of side items and she ate it all. I was most surprised as that is more appetite than I've seen for awhile.

It is now almost 10 p.m. and I have to go back down to check hot packs on pain areas. Then will hit the sack. This may be the most stressful time of my life and demanding. But yet, am learning things I had not known before. Still think I would have made a good doctor.

May go to church tomorrow morning depending. Also tomorrow,

have to get local and federal tax forms finished for Michele as Monday is the deadline. It is also the deadline for our personal Federal, State and Local tax extensions. But will get it done. Really won't take all that much time. The real good news is that our daily trips to hospital are over for now as well as a whole lot of other things that I've been able to get done. So, much relief.

April 14, 1996

Current radiation, shots and trips to hospital done for awhile. Tax deadlines have been met, including going over numbers for Dan, making up returns and extensions for Michele. In other words, I think that I've climbed the mountain and will be doing downhill for awhile. However, still have to go to City of Gahanna to hand carry some tax forms tomorrow, also to hospital to pick up a prescription which contains narcotics. They can not phone or fax it. Boy, what a relief though to be able to back off just a little.

Day wasn't bad although not the 81 degrees we had Friday. Michele has been helpful. Susan brings over a cake or something. Have to put every drug bottle away securely, as Nicholas, one of our grandsons, has a knack of getting into everything he shouldn't. If it's dangerous, he will find it.

One time, I left out a capsule of Cayenne Pepper powder lying on the lazy Susan on the kitchen table. Wouldn't you know that he found it, put it in his mouth and bit into it. We heard him crying and pointing to his mouth. The capsule was there. Luckily, it didn't break open. If it had, don't know what might have happened. His tooth went through the container and just enough got out and it only takes a speck. Don't know of anything that can burn like that stuff. Put together a couple of Easter baskets for Riley, our other grandson, and Nicholas. Riley's response was "Paw Paw, it was sure nice of you to do this for me". He is getting to be a real gentleman.

April 15, 1996

Michele just called and talked for about a half hour. In the process, realized how tired I feel tonight. It's been a long day but I've said that before. Got up this morning, put out trash and after all the usual duties, went to city building and took care of taxes. Then to post office to get several tax envelopes hand stamped with date. Back home-everything still okay, got helper started on outside work, next took off for hospital to pick up prescription for pain pills, went to pharmacy some distance away, then back home.

Got back about noon. Fixed wife a little lunch which was not eaten, ate a bite myself, went out and got chain saw and helper and I cut down two trees. Then chain saw started acting up so went to gas station and bought their best gasoline. Came back and mixed with oil, put in saw and it took off like it didn't know any better. But, it started to rain, then it really came down.

Meantime, went inside to get check book to pay helper and found wife very ill. Was going into shock. Took temperature, blood pressure and pulse, called doctor and finally gave her some grape juice with sugar. She alternated between chills and sweat, but gradually got better. This caused her to become very frightened, which probably amplified her distress. Now about 9:30, will take a bath, shampoo, and stay up until 10 when a pill has to be taken.

April 16, 1996

Today is Meryl's birthday. A lot of company came in. Last person left at 9:40 p.m., end of another long day. However, I think that visitors cheered her up a little and took her mind off the health problem. Am beginning to believe that fear and uncertainty are causing more pain and anxiety than I might have imagined.

Tomorrow, have appointment with oncologist at 1:45. If they give her an IV, probably won't be home until well after 6 p.m. Rented one of two vacant apartments this evening. Had carpet in both cleaned. Was told that it would dry in about an hour but it still felt wet to me. Went down to meet new tenant. Got in bed last night after bath and that is the last thing I can remember until I woke up this morning.

Weather was not all that great. Alternated between rain, sleet, wet snow and a combination of all three. Am beginning to look at different agencies to bring someone in for a little relief. Will know better what to do after the appointment tomorrow. I know there is much to do and much is not getting done.

Every third day, I take pills out of bottles and put them in AM, Noon and PM bags. All this experience is interesting, but it makes me wonder how others in this situation get by. Now, time to hit the sack but forgot to give pain pills for night. Went down and had to wake her up Otherwise, it would have been a difficult night.

April 17, 1996

Had a busy morning and finally got away to doctor about 1 p.m. Arrived just on time. Lab work showed a great reduction in tumor count, in fact, about 75 percent. Dropped from nearly 3500 to just over 700. Also, no weight loss since the last weighing last week. Don't know what the chest X-ray showed as it was taken after the appointment. Perhaps will hear from doctor tomorrow.

April 18, 1996

One of the nicest days so far this year except for wind. Was able to get away for a meeting of the board at the officers' club at the Defense Construction Supply Center. Later went to grocery and spent about $50, including some items I hadn't planned to buy. However, me and sales. Seems that I can't turn down a good bargain. Later, went down to store and picked up some paint for apartments. One couple were both smokers and walls are stained with nicotine. So, have to clean, touch up and some painting except, that Dan has volunteered to do it for me. In fact, when I told him that I would get the trimming done, it upset him.

It's about 9:20 and I've finished most of my requirements for today. Meryl's hair is falling out in bunches now from chemotherapy. That has added a new cleaning problem. Wig people are coming in Saturday morning for a fitting. Meantime, have been calling a few friends as they have been in the dark about what is happening. Several calls tonight and many are shocked at the sudden turn of events.

Biggest problem is a lack of positive attitude. And that, with the anxiety and fear, is what I have always dreaded during a lifetime of smoking. But then, she believes that the nicotine got her through many difficult times. It is extremely difficult for a female spouse to decide between family and career. I know very few women who have been able to end up satisfied with their lives who have tried to do both. Still warm tonight but am not opening a window. Last time it got warm, opened upstairs windows and woke up about 2:30 with stuffed up nostrils. So, that ended the wishful thinking that I am over my sinus infection.

Will do a little work on apartments today and have a meeting of the board of Directors at the Officers' Club at the Defense Supply Center of (DSCC) at 11:30. Also, have to put together instructions on medication, food preparations and possible problems prior to leaving Saturday to deliver speech. Michele and my sister-in-law are filling in for me. It will be a welcome break. So, time now to start medication for today. Both medication and instructions were changed yesterday. Seems that just keeping up with changes is quite a task. The idea is to see what works best. However, the trial and error is a painful process and it seems to me that the medical world ought to have a better handle on what they prescribe.

Have been putting this information into computer and modifying the information as changes occur, then printing new medication schedules.

April 19, 1988

This day started out to be a most trying one until afternoon. Then a change for the better, but have been alternately fresh and tired all day. Talked with the hospital support office today and learned a service is available which provides nurses, therapists, and other support workers. They are to call me. Michele arranged to work at home on some research, so she can stay here while I go to Athens for a meeting at Ohio University.

Have a busy week coming up with a lot scheduled, but don't know that I'll be able to get away. Will probably have to cancel most of events. Friends are staying for awhile Sunday night so that I can go to a dinner with Congressman John Kasick. Don't know it if will work out.

Michele and Susan stopped by again tonight and then went out to dinner. Judge David Johnson, who is Susan's boss, is leaving for Europe shortly, visiting Germany, France and Spain. He will be gone a month. So Susan ought to have an easy time during his absence, with no trials. Dan is coming over tomorrow morning early to paint wall in apartment. I had hoped to help but don't know. Someone is coming to fit Meryl with a wig since the chemo will cause her to lose her hair. Some has come out already. In fact, have to vacuum her bed, to clean up hair she has lost.

April 20, 1996

Was gone yesterday, Saturday, and back Sunday morning. Michele was here when I arrived and sister-in law had already left. Plans to go to Ohio University tomorrow now changed. Everyone had to cancel staying, so I will call early tomorrow and let them know that I can't attend meeting. Perhaps after I talk with the agency tomorrow, I will be able to hire people to help out. Went to Congressman Kasick's dinner tonight. However, friends staying with Meryl had to leave by 7:15 p.m., which I thought would give me plenty of time. But at 7 p.m., when I had planned to leave for home, the dinner hadn't even reached the main course. So I imagine the affair wasn't over until 9 or 9:30. Told Congressman Kasick my situation and why I had to leave. I was seated at the main reserved table right in front of the podium with a number of VIP's including chairman of Republican Party on my right and Kasick to my left. From that position, I was very conspicuous and it was embarrassing to leave, but no choice.

April 21, 1996

Health seems to be improving except for bad pain in right hip, which has just about eliminated any possibility of walking for now. Doctor talks about some radiation on hip but has done nothing. Meryl is in a downstairs bedroom and I am sleeping in our room upstairs. I have set up a phone system so that if anything happens at night, she can push a button and a signal is transmitted. Had to run a special phone line this morning for this. The whole thing only took about an hour.

All is quiet now and when I finish this, will sort out some bills. Have to write checks but will probably do that tomorrow. Anticipate a busy week with daughter gone. Took Michele to airport about 3:30. She has a business trip to Baltimore and will be back Wednesday. She told me that she applied for a six-weeks leave of absence from her company. Am not in favor of that as management does not look favorably on such things, regardless of how valid the reason might be. The condition of her mother is the reason.

Got a call today from Columbus health agency. Was told they had received a call from the hospital to say I needed help with medication and injections. Told her that was all behind for now, and thought they were going to provide help to relieve me and to give her therapy on legs.

Was told that was not part of their service. The spokeswoman was going to call the doctor to see what he had in mind.

I want to find an agency that would provide some relief in chores and time so I can get other work done. Guess will have to wait to see what happens. Am disappointed with follow up on part of all agencies involved, doctors, medical staff, therapists, etc. Am particularly disturbed with lack of coordination between all agencies. When I brought it up with original doctor, was told information was all in computer and it wasn't his fault if others didn't check it. That was a few days after our first visit with him. Haven't seen or heard from him since. The hospital could use a good organizer. Am pretty much convinced that there is little if any communications between the attending physicians.

April 23, 1996

Another long day with a nurse stopping by this afternoon to inform us of services ordered by doctor. Told us that charge would be $91 per visit. Was just out of school. I was surprised at the lack of a professional attitude. Also, had to answer a bunch of questions that I've already answered time after time. It's all in the computer if they would just look. Guess it is easier to ask and it does use up time.

My problem is I don't see a sense of intuitive appreciation. Only sort of a robotic response. That's not the way we used to solve problems. Most of our progress has been because people understood what they were doing rather than just reacting.

Was able to do a couple of errands. Phone was out when I got up. Had to call from a drive-in, and spent nearly 20 minutes accomplishing very little. Phone suddenly became operative about the middle of afternoon.

Phone company said they didn't know why. Said phone was off the hook. At one time, I was in charge of all long distance overseas telephone communications between Belgium and U.S. They don't think I know enough to figure out a simple telephone problem.

Made some lentil soup which I served for supper. Was pretty good, even if I do say so. Had two helpings. Meryl had a bad evening even though most of day was pretty good. In spite of gravity of health problem, she has been smoking again. I have suspected. This is happening in the bathroom with the window open so we won't be able to smell tobacco smoke. What is it about cigarettes that holds some people even though they are in a life threatening situation? I had been sort of positive about the future, but knowing the habit has not changed, my confidence has diminished. Worse, she is not telling the doctor the truth either.

Dan says that at this point, it doesn't make any difference, anyhow. I disagree for a number of reasons. It is now fairly late in the evening, as she was in so much pain and nausea that I stayed up with her to make certain I could help with whatever she needed. It's tough to just sit there while all that suffering goes on. But using a special salve and hot compresses covered with towels seem to provide a great deal of relief.

April 26, 1996

Meryl had a fairly decent day, in fact the best in several weeks. Think that an adjustment in pain medication and timing on nausea pills is mostly responsible. Picked up Michele at airport tonight about 6:40. Had planned a salad, macaroni & cheese and fish sticks for supper. My homemade salad dressing has now become a fixture. Nobody wants anything else. So she stayed for supper and all that was prepared was eaten. Being a full time cook has brought back a lot of memories about the days when I helped my parents when I was young. Funny how it seems like yesterday and yet, the very far distant past. Susan left a message while I was at the airport. Her mother was taken to the hospital today with internal bleeding. They will do test tomorrow.

This is getting tough on Dan. He was kind of shook up when I talked with him a short time ago. He closes on the sale of his former home Friday. That will be a relief. His temporary tenant moved out last weekend, so timing was perfect.

April 27, 1996

Got up early and the new nurse service started again. Found out that nurse has been out of school only about a month so she has had no experience. Doctor wanted me to check as he wanted an experienced nurse. He also told me yesterday over telephone that he would be in San Francisco, leaving today and back next Tuesday. Gave me his motel phone number in case I needed to reach him.

The doctor had returned my call from yesterday but, when I called back, he had already left home. His wife told me he would telephone her about 10 p.m. and she would have him call me. When he reached me, we chatted nearly 30 minutes about medication and other issues. A few of his comments disturbed me quite a bit. He is concerned about cancer spreading to more spinal areas, and that would be the worst of all situations.

Not a good day, same as the weather. If we could have a little sunshine, I think everybody would cheer up. Sometimes I wonder if this is our reward for years of strife and turmoil. However, there are many great memories and those overcome the things we may not have liked.

April 28, 1996

This newly-commissioned nurse with no uniform comes only on Monday and Thursday, and only to draw blood. So she is only here a very short time. Some relief, in that we don't have to go to clinic or hospital to get blood work done.

The doctor earlier had asked me to see if she was experienced with cancer patients. When he gets back, will have to tell him the facts. She was somewhat put out that he wanted a copy of test results given to me. She said most doctors don't want their patients to see that information. However, they will be mailed to me.

If there is a problem, I'll let the doctor straighten it out. Don't understand this attitude that patients aren't allowed to see their records. Mexico is just the opposite. You don't have to ask for copies. That's automatic. In addition, the doctor goes over the test results and compares them with previous tests. He also explains each item as he goes down through the list.

Winds have been terrible and keep blowing down trees and limbs. It also blew off a large shutter and broke a red bud tree in two down at the apartments. Can't remember having so much wind damage. Am now worried about a couple of large trees that would fall into the house if they came down. May have them cut down at a cost of about $1,000 per tree. Seems that there would be many cords of firewood at about $90 per cord. But you have to be in the business and I don't have time.

Tomorrow, sister-in-law is coming in morning. I will try to get a number of chores done, including welding on the mower and a whole lot of shopping.

* * *

DAILY RECORDS III

April 29, 1996

Sister-in-law got here about 10:15 or so this morning. Since Dan was doing something else at that point, went down to apartment and repaired fan in bedroom that had gotten loose. Had to make a part to overcome the problem. Got back home and Dan had called and said he would arrive in a half hour. Then the phone rang and it was Susan. She was locked out of the house and Nicholas was in bed upstairs. Dan did not have his car phone turned on so she couldn't reach him. So got in car, drove out. When I arrived, she had found a door that had been left open. Lost about an hour in the process.

Dan was waiting when I got back and we went out to pick up a couch from Meryl's office. Was really heavy and was surprised that the two of us could handle it. In the process, sort of turned my left ankle so it's a little sore. By the time all this was done, it was nearly 3:30.

Sister-in-law agreed to stay but had to leave by 5:30. So, went shopping, but not too successful, too much traffic and not enough time. Did pick up a foam rubber pad for Meryl's bed. It really made a huge difference in comfort. I was gratified that I had thought to do this.

Have decided that frying in a typical fry pan needs to be thought about. Why not a deeper pan so that grease does not fly all over the place. When I was out today, looked at a set of pans on sale but decided to look some more. Don't need any more fry pans and two of them came with the set. There was a beautiful heavy stainless steel set that I would have purchased several years ago but cleaning is always a problem. So either stoneware or Teflon is the way to go when one does as much special cooking as I am these days. Cooked up some vegetable soup for supper along with grilled cheese sandwiches. Amazing just how much the art of cooking evolves in dire circumstances.

April 30, 1996

Didn't make it to church this morning. Was a little sore from over-doing it yesterday and ankle was sore. However, put on shoes that gave extra support and not bad now. Seems there are a million things to do constantly around here. Had company at noon who stayed about an hour.

Finally got down to rented apartment about 2:30 and was able to spend about an hour. It is now all finished. Touched up bad spots with paint, finished two bad places in ceiling that I had to tape and spackle and spotted with paint, reglued loose wall paper plus a few more odds and ends. Made some adjustments on furnace and the place now is ready for new tenants. Stopped at other apartment which still had some work to do and left ladder so all will be there first chance I have to get that one finished.

Michele stopped by tonight. Left about 8 p.m. She is leaving for Minneapolis tomorrow morning. Will be back Tuesday. All is now put away, wife's in bed and I'm about to do the same. And it isn't even 9:00 p.m. yet. Tomorrow, will get in touch with some of the agencies which provide home help. Guess it isn't covered by insurance but at least, it's deductible as medical expense.

Still do not have results of blood tests from last week. If I do not have them by Wednesday am going to talk with doctor and get someone else to handle this matter. Am tired of hearing how we shouldn't be seeing these results, which we are apt to misinterpret and do the wrong thing. So much for letting off that round of steam.

Susan's mother was taken to the hospital with a bleeding ulcer. Had to give her two pints of blood. Now back home. Talked with her tonight but they are not giving her the medical treatment that is being used by some doctor's. They told her that a bacteria was not the cause of an ulcer. They also told her that they didn't know what caused hers.

I once stated that a general's lot in life was to clear up what is confused and confuse what is clear. But then, am I not doing just that?

About three years or so ago, Dan's dog, Sundance, contracted lung cancer and had to be put to sleep. I wrote him a letter trying to comfort him a little and in the beginning, told him that all of us, Susan, his Mom, myself were all feeling his sorrow. Completely left out Michele who was in California and didn't even know what had happened.

And the thought that I had left her out was probably based upon the fact that she didn't know. However, should have stated something to clarify.

We were talking about that situation the other night and asked Michele if she had ever seen the letter. She said, "what letter", so I printed out a copy. She caught the omission immediately and let me know about it. Then, she wanted a copy of the letter so I told her I would print a better copy. Very quickly added her name and printed that for her. She was surprised and believe it or not, pleased. Sometimes even I am amazed at how careful we must be in everything we do, no matter how good the intentions.

May 1, 1996

Not too good a day for patient. Much nausea and pills didn't seem to do much good. Not too surprised though with all the radiation she has gotten. Nausea is a symptom of radiation exposure if it is of any significance.

Tomorrow is Dan's 40th birthday and I find it hard to believe that all those years have gone already. Seems like only yesterday that he was growing up. Michele will be 42 later this month although she looks more like 30. Susan is having a party for Dan Sunday night and has invited 50 people or so. Dan is not real happy with all this, with the problems. Her mother is still not over the bleeding ulcer and had to have two pints of blood while in the hospital.

Got my part back for tractor this afternoon so will try to get it on sometime soon. Michele got back from Minneapolis last night feeling under the weather and stayed home today with an upset stomach. Seems to be going around, but what isn't with this crazy weather.

The joy of challenge is not to be set aside. This has been one of those days in which I wonder where it went and where, I know not. Had an appointment this morning about 9:30 here at home, then Meryl had a couple of visitors who stayed nearly half hour. About 11:30, health service sent a dietitian out to talk, you guessed it, about diet and food. Some of the things she told us were the exact opposite of what others have told us. And as usual, our great American medical world is out of contact with each other.

Meryl placed an order for supper which really surprised me. She had been eating just bits and pieces. Tonight, the order was for mashed potatoes, broiled pork chop and a special slaw based on a recipe that

Susan's mother has. So, got the recipe, went to the grocery store, then came home and prepared mashed potatoes, (first time I've ever made mashed potatoes) broiled two pork chops, made the slaw and served a gourmet dinner fit for a king or queen or whomever. This is the first time she has eaten this much in at least three months, and she cleared her plate.

May 2, 1996

Nurse came in this morning but no copies of tests. Later in afternoon, got dressed and went to luncheon for Gen. Colin Powell. Got there too late for private reception because of complications at home. Did get there in time for lunch and his speech which was attended by about three thousand people.

Michele is down with flu, which seems to have descended upon this area. This one does not go away overnight but from what I have heard, lingers for three or four days. Am washing my hands at least 15 times everyday. I have a scheduled speech at Ohio University a week from tomorrow night. The announcements and program have been published and gone out. There must be a way for relief so I can attend. All the agencies with whom I've talked said they would call me back with more info but have not heard from any of them. After lunch today, Dan was here and he stayed all afternoon. Said he wanted to spend part of his birthday with his Mom. Also picked up his presents which he didn't expect.

While he was here, I went to nearby blood lab and obtained results of all bloodwork done so far. They have agreed to give me copies so won't have to argue with anyone any longer.

May 3, 1996

Virus that is going around is of the 48 hour variety and some offices in Columbus have half the people off. Real problem is that we can't have unnecessary exposure because of wife's lowered immunity condition. I even spray the house after visitors.

Susan and Nicholas stopped by tonight. He had a runny nose and I wouldn't let him get within 10 feet of Meryl. Then sprayed after they left. Explained to Susan outside. Would you believe that as we talked, it started to rain. She took time to smell the blooming lilacs anyway. Susan had asked Meryl to come to surprise party for Dan. I was able to get away for about two hours this afternoon and got a lot done.

May 4, 1996

Guess Dan's birthday party went okay. Michele called to ask if I wanted to go over, but told her I couldn't. She offered to come over. Told her the danger of exposure remained, whether she stayed all night or just a short time. Dan got to party about hour and a half late. The guys who were supposed to have him there at 5 p.m. did not keep their commitment, although Dan might have had something to do with that.

Meryl is in bed, I'm upstairs doing daily memo and as soon as this is finished, will hit the sack. Don't know why I am tired or perhaps it's only the frustration. Wife continues to have severe leg pains. Now have three heating pads in order to cover all areas of pain. Each night, I put hot towels on both legs, then covered them with dry towels after I had put a special salve on her legs. After about fifteen minutes, the pain seems to subside and she is able to go to sleep. Not sure whether the treatment or the pain pills bring the relief, but the combination works and that is all that is important.

May 5, 1996

Got up about 6:45, did a few things and got ready to go to church. First, took care of medication, etc. Was gone about forty-five minutes which seems to be the limit to being away. Was back before 9 and took care of breakfast, pills, etc. There are before meal pills and after meal pills.

Had a few minutes so packed up computer equipment that IRS will pick up sometime tomorrow. I have been a volunteer for the IRS for years doing taxes for people with low incomes. This year, the IRS asked me to head up an electronic filing system in Columbus. Picked up the equipment in Cincinnati but will not be able to make trip to return it because of circumstances. So one of their agents is coming to Columbus tomorrow to get it. Was going to do some paper work but that got sidetracked. Sister-in-law came out, cooked noodles and a roast after I had gone to grocery to pick up a list that was needed. Yard helper showed up at 11 so I let him start on a couple of things at apartments.

Next, decided to go from winter to summer. Took off flannel sheets and replaced with regular ones. So as far as I'm concerned, the seasons have changed. Will probably feel strange.

Didn't get much of anything done rest of day except go over tax matters with Michele, who dropped by in the afternoon. She left about 6 p.m., suddenly remembering she had an appointment. We never seem to have enough time to finalize anything.

Am starting to realize that I'm beginning to become somewhat stressed out. Now beginning the fourth month since original diagnosis. Am going to have to start thinking about what I have to do to maintain my strength and physical condition. Will have to discipline myself to get the things done that I need. Am going to force myself to a program of at least half hour a day of some kind of physical exercise.

May 6, 1996

Went to spouse's office this morning and she went along. First time in several weeks she has been able to walk, albeit with a walker. Nausea is major problem most of the time and am sure that radiation and chemo have caused that.

Didn't get much done today or, rather, not what I had planned to do. Helper showed up, but I had him work alone. Short order cook that I've become, prepared corn on the cob, noodles, roast beef and strawberries for dinner. Can't believe it but she cleaned the entire plate.

Nurse got blood this morning. I asked her some questions about blood test verbiage but she said she just didn't remember. Said it was in a book and she would bring it for me the next time she came. Could not believe a graduate, registered nurse giving an answer like that. Goes back to my speech in Washington about eight years ago when I said mediocrity must never become the standard for excellence. Perhaps ignorance has become the standard for mediocrity. If this happened to me, I would blush, if that is possible.

May 7, 1996

Appointment with oncologist today at 1 p.m. Lab work first so had to get there by 12:30. Got a look at latest X-rays and there have been a lot of them. Doctor indicates that she is making good progress. I still am on pins and needles, and will be.

His records were out where I could look at them. I found a letter he had written stating that he felt the typical patient with lung cancer such as Meryl's has a life expectancy of four to eleven months, with less than five percent surviving for two years. The shock of seeing this will stay with me, but will keep it from her.

This weather has now gotten me to a point where I may just tear out what little hair I have left. My helper showed up and he finished clearing out weed areas except for one. Then we cut down the tree we didn't finish a couple of weeks ago because it started raining. This took about an hour and was a much more difficult job than I had assumed. Next, cut down what was left of Red Bud which the wind had snapped in two.

From there, helper wanted me to fix the seat in his car which took another hour. Next, took out the new mower and started it so he could get trimming at apartments done. This mower has enough horse power to cut through tall weeds. Best cutting mower I've ever had. In about fifteen minutes it started to rain, then pour. Had to quit and put it off. Now have some grass that is over twelve inches tall. And the grass hasn't been dry for over three weeks now.

Caught up on part of paper work. Went to store and then came back and fixed supper. Easy tonight as all I did was warm up mashed potatoes, noodles, etc., which turned out to be fine. Desert was wafers and sliced Red Delicious apple. Called Ohio University ROTC and told them I would make it for speech Friday night. Dan is going to stay until I get back. Found out that OU president as well as other VIP's will also be there so speech will have to be extra good.

They had contacted another general in case they would need a backup for me. He called and had to back out. So they were relieved when I told them I was coming, God Willing and the Creek don't rise no higher. Still have to repair tractor, mower is welded so that is OK. Was going to do that today but too wet and cool.

May 8, 1996

Got a little work done this morning but had to leave for doctor's about 11:45. Got there at 12:25 or five minutes early. Lab work consisted of taking blood and a chest X-ray. Blood is improving after reaching a low that had me a little concerned. Doctor says that tumor has reduced.

The X-ray shows the tumor in right lung that has gone from a solid mass to one that is now broken up into many smaller pieces.

Started new round of chemo today and she elected to take via an IV. Seems the effects are much easier to take that way than with the capsules. However, for the next four days, she gets three capsules each day. If it gets to be too much, the doctor said she could come back and take treatments via IV everyday if she wanted.

By the time she was finished today, and stopped to pick up four new prescriptions at almost $2,000, it was after 6 p.m. She had noodles and corn on the cob for supper. Had a tornado warning until 10 p.m. Storm has passed over and is now about 30 miles east of here. The sirens have been blaring constantly since 8:45.

May 9, 1996

Patient had terrible day. I found it very stressful. It's difficult to watch all that suffering and unable to do anything about it. She was able to take the chemo pills, although it was questionable whether I would have to take her back to get it by IV.

The nausea really came back today and was that way from about 11 a.m. on. Very little, or practically no food as it didn't look like it would stay down.

Started out by working on mower. Everything went fine and was just about finished when I was called. Thought it would take only a couple of minutes to finish but no such luck. So went in and found spouse in terrible nausea. Called doctor and did what he told me. After giving her the medication, she became almost as though she had taken dope.

Read the pharmacist's print out on the medication and found that she was having practically every side effect possible. She went to bed about 6 p.m., and has slept most of the time since.

Meantime, I spent almost all afternoon trying to write speech for tomorrow night. Could only write perhaps ten minutes at a time without interruption. It is difficult to maintain a train of thought that way, so it took a couple of hours.

Then, took a few minutes and went out and worked on the mower again. This time, found the problem and fixed it. So now, believe am ready to mow if time is ever available. This is one of those days when I think the nurse is physically not well. But I will survive, I guess.

217

Michele says I look skinny. Weigh about 153 which is about where I like to be but apparently, everyone is used to my being heavier.

I think one of the problems with many who retire is that they lose a sense of accomplishment. That reduces their sense of esteem and self appreciation, and they perhaps gain a sense that they no longer have a useful function in their lives. While I have never felt this way, the responsibilities I now have would certainly negate any feelings of that sort.

May 10, 1996

I pumped up with three cups of coffee after speech in Athens so I probably won't be able to go to sleep before 4 a.m. Had rain going and coming, but not too bad. Speech seemed to go well, and Ohio University president asked for copy of speech.

His wife Renee was very gracious with her compliments and asked me how one person could assemble so much on the subject of leadership. She said that while she was somewhat conversant with the subject, she had never heard so much that applied and wanted to know how I had learned so much. Told her that I was a good listener. She had a dubious look so I mentioned that my Dad had once told me that if you "Only talk and never listen, you are limited to what you already know."

Dr. Robert Glidden heard me. He commented I had a number of good one liners and he especially liked that one. He wants to use some of them. I said that I would send him a copy. It won't include everything because in between lines, added whatever came to mind.

Had some fun at the beginning as I acknowledged VIP's, etc. The wife of the colonel, Professor of Military Science of the Reserve Officer Training Corps, was from Germany, as were some of her family, and they were all together at one table. So when I finished all the acknowledgments, I looked at the table and said, this is for the special edification of a small group assembled at the table directly in front of the head table.

So I said - "Meine Dammen und Herren or my ladies and gentlemen." Then added a few more words in German. Amazing how quickly you are accepted when you speak the other person's language. Finally was able to leave about 11:05. Program was long and delayed. Didn't give speech until about 10:00.

When I got home, both Dan and Riley were asleep. Had taken care of all medication before I left except what was needed at bedtime. Had that out so Dan would have no problem. She was asleep. Dan got Riley up and they went home. Nothing as heartwarming as a small child who has been awakened at 1 a.m. I just hate to see that, but they get over it quickly and soon forget. This should test our memories.

May 11, 1996

Today was the fourth day of current chemo, with tomorrow yet to go. That will complete this phase. This time is much worse than the first. There has been constant nausea and she is not eating enough to keep a mouse alive.

Am really a little worried about whether chemo is damaging the liver. This stuff is plain poison and attacks both good and bad. Add the maximum radiation she has already had, and it takes a lot to survive just the treatment. Also, have a great deal of concern about the fact that treatment is drastically reducing her immune system.

Helper got a lot of mowing done yesterday and I was going to finish up today but it rained all day. The creek that goes through the west side of my property looks like a river.

Several days ago, while going for a prescription, I hit a chuck hole with the right front wheel. However, I didn't realize that any damage had occurred until Dan noticed when I started to leave last night for Ohio University that the hub cap was missing on that wheel.

Looking closer, we noticed that the rim was damaged and the tire seemed to have a bulge. So drove another car rather than take a chance of a problem on the road. Called the garage to see how much a new rim would be would be and was told about $208 or so, depending upon exactly which rim.

Called an auto salvage place, they had one left in stock and the price was $35. Could not get away long enough to pick it up so perhaps Monday will be able to do so. However, looked again at the damaged rim and I might be able to straighten it out. Also, forgot to get a price on a hub cap because even though I remember very vividly hitting the chuck hole, can't remember where it was.

Did get a few more things done today including some special wiring which I had to finish by Monday. Down-spout is finished, more hand mowing is done, tractor is now ready to go, paper work is close to being caught up so what am I fretting about. Guess it's just that the tension never ceases. I also got to the grocery today, while sister-in-law and niece stopped by and stayed with Meryl.

May 12, 1996

Meryl has not been out of bed since Thursday, except to go to the bathroom, and is eating even less. Didn't cook anything today. Dan and Susan went to a friend's house, then to see Susan's mother, and stopped here late this afternoon. Michele had been here an hour, arriving at 3 p.m. That gave me time for a couple of errands, was back about 4:10. Other than making copies of some medical records, real purpose of trip was to pick up Michele's birthday present. In the space of an hour, drove about 22 miles and made two stops.

Michele talked with doctor while I was gone. He wants me to bring Meryl in tomorrow about 1 p.m. Am to call and make arrangements.

She is very weak and tired, in addition to the intense nausea from chemo. She finished this round today and she was able to keep pills down. Neupogen shots begin Tuesday for ten days. Each shot which I will give her is $138 or $1380 for the ten shots. This will be the second round. A new problem has shown itself, an intense burning sensation. Doctor thinks it may be nerve damage from radiation. Probably change medication tomorrow, again. Now have a whole bag full of bottles of unused medication. If this keeps up, one day will be able to fill prescriptions from medication on hand.

* * *

DAILY RECORD IV

May 13, 1996

Took Meryl to office this morning for an appointment with doctor. After examination, he decided to put her in the hospital as she had deteriorated terribly after last round of chemo. It was several hours before arrangements were completed. We left for hospital in afternoon, finalized admission red tape and finally got her into a room. Almost immediately, people began to pop in asking all kinds of questions about medication, history, etc. If anyone pretends there is any semblance of coordination and communications between the various entities who are involved, then my experience through life has been too demanding. How can one doctor send his patient to be hospitalized without sending along all the necessary information. And if he did all this, then the people on the other end didn't bother familiarizing themselves with that information. I would say that at least two hours were wasted because of all the questions. Finally about 9 p.m., I decided to go home while Michele stayed at the hospital overnight. If I had any faith in the medical profession, this experience pretty well reduced it to nothing more than an idea. I am very apprehensive about the competency of those who are treating her and even more so about the future.

It seems that after a lifetime of concern, work and stress, we should be able to look back, appreciate that which is behind us and look forward to each new day as a fulfillment of all that past effort. That's not the way it is. Won't know until Wednesday just what the rest of the week holds.

May 14, 1996

Somehow, the dawn and a bright sun change one's outlook considerably. Was tired, perhaps more so than I thought last night with a frame of mind that did not support the physical and mental deficiencies. Woke up at 6 a.m. with a bright sun. Yesterday, doctor put Meryl in hospital to counter dehydration and other problems resulting from last round of chemo. Meryl called from hospital this morning, said they had her up until midnight with a Magnetic Resolution Image (MRI) at 10 p.m.

Doctors asked questions for two hours. It seems no matter what is on the computer or how many times the routine questions are asked, it still goes on. Told one intern yesterday after he asked questions for 20 minutes that if I ever have to go to hospital, I will make 50 copies of answers and hand them out. His answer - It wouldn't do any good because they would ask the questions anyway. When I asked him what purpose it served, he stated the record was important. But he did not take any notes.

Meryl also said in the telephone conversation they awakened her this morning at 5 a.m., but at 8:50 a.m. they still had not brought her breakfast. Seems that her floor is last on the list. So wonder if they get lunch in time for supper.

May 15, 1996

Today was a little different than the days recently gone by. Perhaps a little less stressful also. Got up, got a few things done at home, got a call from Meryl at 8:50 a.m., saying again they had gotten her up at 5 a.m., given her pain and nausea medicine and continuing IV's. She was really hungry, and they still hadn't brought breakfast.

However, I couldn't believe the difference in her condition in just one day in the hospital. She had a full breakfast of scrambled eggs, bacon and juice. I went to the hospital about 10:30 a.m., and she was feeling much better. Dan had just gotten there. We really didn't have a chance to say much because there was constant traffic of doctors, nurses, aids, psychologists, and therapists. I think someone was in or out about every five minutes. I noticed that her hand was swelling where the IV needle was inserted. Called for help and finally had to go out and do a little foot-putting-down to get someone. Sister-in- law came in about 12:30, then Michele about 2 p.m. I wanted to get the rest of the grass knocked down if possible today because it was fairly dry but possibility of rain tomorrow. Left about 3 p.m. stated mowing, made a few phone calls. Finished right at 6 p.m., cleaned up, opened mail and called hospital.

Michele suggested I not go back to the hospital, but relax and get a full night's sleep. She said she would stop by about 7:30 after leaving the hospital, so I invited her to go out for dinner. She accepted, except she grabbed the check and paid the bill. Brother Bill called after I arrived home and asked about Meryl. He didn't know that anything was wrong. We have not told many people, but word has gotten around.

May 18, 1996

It's warm right now as I write this in an upstairs room. Would have been nice to have a few days of spring before summer arrived. Just back from Ft. Knox where I am a member of the retiree advisory board. Left Thursday as wife was feeling much better and still in hospital. It is now Saturday.

Arrived home about 10:55 a.m. and called Michele. No answer, so called hospital and guess that I awakened Meryl. Dan was there and he brought me up to date on what happened while I was gone. Seems that radiologist misread X-ray and announced that tumor has greatly increased. This prompted additional X-rays, Cat Scan, Lumbar tap, and other tests.

Then, radiologist told doctor he had misread X-ray, and tumor had actually shrunk about fifty percent. All the tests were clear, so putting her through all that was unnecessary. Dan said he was leaving to prepare for a small birthday party for his son Riley. Told him I would be out sometime in the afternoon, and that I had found set of BDU's (battle dress uniform) for Riley in a store near Ft. Knox. It might be a little large, I said, but should be okay.

Later, went to hospital and found wife asleep. She woke up for a second to say, "Hi", and back to sleep. I sat down in an easy chair and dozed for about an hour.

Woke up about 2:45 when she had to go to bathroom. Aide came in and changed bed linen while she was out of bed. Lots of company coming in so guess she is sleeping in between times. Left about 3:00 and went to Dan's. Gave Riley his outfit, stayed about an hour and half, then came home. Michele was going to hospital to spend the night with Meryl. She thought I should go home and get some rest.

She had talked with Meryl who also felt I should not return to hospital. So, came home, caught up on unpacking, paper work, and it is now just 9 p.m. Dusk has arrived with another hot day predicted for tomorrow. For some reason, have felt all day that it was Sunday. Will try mowing sometime during the day tomorrow. That should make grass manageable again.

Have not written about days while I was gone. Neupogen shots were stopped in my absence as white blood count had jumped well above normal. Other than the unnecessary procedures as a result of the misreading of X-ray, patient seems to be feeling much better. However, the critical period is coming up when her red counts and white counts will drop. This, as I understand, may necessitate a transfusion and perhaps even a transfusion of platelets. Am very apprehensive about the transfusion, as I have very little confidence in how well the blood is tested before it is used. It is not just the transmittal of AIDS, but other diseases as well. Who knows whether the blood contains other types of cancer. Am assured that all is fine but have seen too many mistakes.

The nurses and aides on duty have been tremendous, extremely dedicated. I couldn't ask more. A medical student, Robin, has been especially helpful. A therapist promised all sorts of things, but usually has not followed up, so am disappointed. But most of all, my disappointment is with the lack of any coordinated effort. Also at times, doctors do not seem to realize the effect negative statements have on the patients.

Can't shake the feeling that if something happens early on, it will be the treatment that caused it, rather than the cancer. But what can I do?

May 19, 1996

Michele called and said she would be going to hospital shortly, so I went with her. We didn't leave until late. It was a bad day. Doctor told Meryl at 5:30 that temperature was up, she was having a drastic drop in white blood cells. She was barely able to breath with difficulty. Michele and I got her calmed down, found girl medical student Robin whom I like so well and had her explain what was going on.

When Meryl finally settled down to where she was no longer in panic, they gave her some kind of drug. She acted as though she had consumed three or four martinis. No breakfast, two spoonfuls of macaroni and cheese, and that was her food for the day by the time we left. Had her back on IV with antibiotic. Drug finally was beginning to wear off as we left.

Forecast is for five straight days of 80-90 degree weather, then back to 60's or in that vicinity. Bedroom was hot last night even with open windows. Finally turned on window unit, got room cool in about 30 minutes, then turned it off and went to sleep. Sort of planned to start today by going to Mass this morning but got up a little later than expected, used up an hour and by that time, did not have enough time to get ready to go.

Later came home from hospital, changed, gassed tractor and started mowing. It was slow and after two hours, was not even half finished. Then tractor engine started to act up so had to quit. Will have to see what is wrong. It was acting as though it was running only on one cylinder. May be a burned out spark plug cable. So, cleaned up, had a light supper. Dan and Susan now are at the hospital. I hope they will call me to let me know what is happening when they get home.

May 20, 1996

Air conditioning system was not working properly in hospital and it was cold. Meryl was made comfortable, and I finally got a blanket from a nurse. I kept it over my shoulders until middle of afternoon when system started warming up. Stayed at hospital until about 5 p.m. when Michele came in. Dan stopped by for a couple of minutes, then had to leave to pick up boys. Dan's wife Susan, a court bailiff, had a jury deliberating and didn't know when she would be able to leave.

Michele called about fifteen minutes ago from her home, and told me she was going back to hospital to stay all night. Guess neither she nor Meryl wanted me to do this. Doctor came in tonight and said that they were going to feed her intravenously to try to get her built up. I felt this was needed for some time, but guess Meryl reacted as though it was another blow. When Michele called, I asked her to stop by and I would go with her. Apparently they were concerned about my health. Think I would be more comfortable there but resigned to staying home.

During my stay at the hospital earlier today, I did some reading, took a little nap and, except for walking the hall three or four times, just sat in a chair most of the time I was there. Have to confess this kind of inactivity is not exactly good for me. About time to set up an exercise regimen to make up for the inactivity of the body and the stress of the mind.

Received a letter today from Dr. Jaime Narvaez in Juarez, Mexico. He was the staff doctor in the clinic where my wife was a patient. I had sent him the latest blood results, biopsy report, and other data. His letter was quite detailed with suggestions of changing supplements to meet the new conditions. It was so detailed that he must have spent quite a bit of time going over everything. Wish the medical world here in the states would take some lessons. From what Michele told me, and she just called from hospital, this feeding will continue at home after discharge, depending on what happens. Guess someone will come out each night and then again in the morning. This upset spouse because whoever it is that will do this came in tonight and told her he would rather put a tube through the rectum and feed directly into the stomach. Michele told him that was not the doctor's instructions and she wished he hadn't brought this up. Said he felt it was his duty to do so. I get the feeling we are dealing with machines. Worse, everyone acts independently and I don't know of any overall plan of treatment. As far as I'm concerned, this is a total nightmare. Are we doing the right thing? I am very concerned that we are not.

May 21, 1996

Just got home from hospital where I have been all day. Was raining when I left house this morning about 9:30. Morning started badly with all counts down very low, fear of infection because of low immunity, red count down so low that they decided on transfusion. One packet was completed by the time I left with another still to come. Michele came in and will stay the night. However, temperature is down and Meryl is alert again. Blood pressure is back to normal, no side effects. Coming to the end of the critical period for this round of chemo. If all goes as expected, things should turn around. Hoping this will end the bad nights resulting from taking her near death and bringing her back. Dan just called from his car. He was on his way to get a bite to eat after finishing teaching his law classes. He starts a trial tomorrow morning in Urbana, Ohio, which is in Champaign, County. We won't see him for a few days.

The young female medical student who has been so great has gone home. Her sister who had just graduated from college was killed in an automobile accident so she will be gone for a week. Such a tragedy shouldn't have to happen. Will write a note to her to see if I can reduce some of her pain. A doctor who has a high position with the hospital stopped in this afternoon for a few minutes. Didn't recognize him at first and then realized who he was. That visit did not go without the staff on duty noticing. And the word will get around to the doctors. Anyway, it was nice of him. Haven't seen or talked with him for awhile. Getting late and even though I've done little or nothing today, seem to be tired.

May 22, 1996

Long day and little if anything accomplished. Possibility that wife will be released tomorrow. If so, it will be because of the complications of staying more than ten days or that is what I understand. She will have to stay on IV's for awhile and they are sending equipment to the house. Have been told that they will teach me what to do. Actually, if she starts eating full meals again, this won't be necessary. While she is eating more again and numbers are starting to come up, I've seen many mistakes that have been made simply because numbers are not being watched closely enough. The first time around, when potassium, magnesium, etc., got low, I just gave her some supplements that brought numbers back. In the hospital, they seem to wait until numbers become critical and then start remedial action too late. At least, that is the way it strikes me.

May 23, 1996

I spent practically all day at the hospital so didn't get much of outdoors. However, my niece came in about 6 p.m. and was staying until Michele got there. Blood work shows that everything is beginning to come back. However, platelets had dropped to a real danger point so they started her on another transfusion tonight. This time, they are putting in only platelets and antibiotics. Danger cycle of four days or so after chemo is coming to end, so each day should show improvement until time for next round. If there is not a complete recovery, including the strength to be self-sufficient, don't believe that we will allow next chemo round that is due in about 3 weeks. If all goes well, this hospital stay may end in a day or so, depending upon what happens. One question I keep asking myself is that if chemotherapy keeps destroying the immune system, does it destroy the body's ability to assist in fighting the cancer. Few, if any, want to answer that question.

When I arrived home after my day at the hospital, I picked up a couple more parts for mower and tractor and just finished repairs. Problem was that mosquitoes were thicker than blazes even though I was inside carriage house. But, had doors open and lights on so guess that attracted them. So got my spray can and kept spraying and they kept coming in and I kept on spraying and they kept on coming in...well now, that could be a never ending dissertation. Believe that I found trouble with tractor engine.

May 24, 1996

Received a telephone call early this morning saying Meryl was coming home today. I got to the hospital as early as possible and had a conference with the doctor's nurse at 11:20 a.m. She said all that was needed was the doctor's release. We waited, and waited, and waited. I think everyone on duty was embarrassed. A female doctor finally came in about 6 p.m. to go over new instructions. She wrote up over fifteen prescriptions, part of which I will fill in the morning. The pharmacy closed at 6 p.m. The rest I will have filled at Wright-Patterson AFB next week. If they would just write these in advance, I could take advantage of my military privileges. That is about the only medical benefit retired military people have these days. Of course, the privileges of shopping at the Post Exchanges and Commissaries are still available. Also had to buy a bedside potty. I left about 6:20 and drove about two miles away. A few pieces of pipe, a seat and a bucket totaled $90. The rental, if I didn't want to purchase, was $30 per month. Got back to hospital about 7 p.m., and Meryl was released to leave.

Arrived home about 8:10 p.m., after spending practically the entire day just waiting. The female doctor was most apologetic and tried to cooperate. The young nurse on duty was literally beside herself and took it on herself to give all necessary medication as well as shot.

Dan and Michele were both here when we arrived home. Dan just left about 20 minutes ago. Will have to get prescriptions filled first thing tomorrow, as most of medication is all new. Think I have enough unused medicine to start a pharmacy. Also have to update my sheet of when prescriptions are to be given. Have more duties now, but won't be spending entire days at hospital. Dan and Michele are taking more responsibility. Michele has gotten permission to work twenty hours a week until the situation changes. Also, therapist and a nurse each come in three times a week. Still trying to find someone willing to spend a few hours each day.

Received an invitation from former Governor James Rhodes inviting me to a dinner for his former cabinet members on June 6. Michele is going to stay with Meryl so I can go. Also, found a message on recorder asking if I would take part in a briefing for the assistant secretary of defense on June 12 in Washington. Two hours have been set aside so it will be a one day trip or back by evening. Last time I briefed the secretary of army, he had set aside 45 minutes and we didn't finish up until over four hours later. Caused us to miss the flight back and had to order a small twin engine army plane to pick up Dr. Charles Ping, the president of Ohio University and myself. We were presenting an experimental program I had formulated at Ohio University to bring back army ROTC.

May 25, 1996

Have no speeches planned this year for the 4th of July for the first time in many years. Felt it best to cancel everything except for a few commitments.

Started out this morning by getting to pharmacy just when they opened. Dismissal from hospital last night was too late to get prescriptions. Got there at 9 a.m., and it took over an hour and twenty minutes to fill them. That was not because they were busy or prescriptions were complicated.

Medications came to well over $1,000 with my share being about $82. The female doctor agreed to give me duplicates on all the prescriptions yesterday so will plan to go to Wright-Pat sometime in the next week or so. Michele has agreed to stay while I'm gone. Doctor canceled the IV plan at home, saying that risk of infection was the reason. So that is one task that I will not have to take on. However, with release, three more Neupogen shots have to be given with first one this evening. Then one more for each of next two days. And I end up with over $1,000 of the serum left in the refrigerator. That's because they gave her so much medication in the hospital. After getting all the medicine home this morning, went outside and took care of a number of chores I had been putting off. Finally back about 2:30 at which time Susan came in, and I went with Michele to look at a car for her. They both took off later, as they are going out tonight for Michele's birthday, which is tomorrow. Fixed macaroni and cheese for supper plus fruit Jello, which was much more than I thought Meryl would eat. Yet, she cleared the plate and really surprised me. About an hour ago, she had some Fritos and chocolate ice cream, not to mention a whole slew of pills. Then to bed and except for a little pain in legs, was feeling much better.

May 26, 1996

Did not go to church this morning as couldn't leave. Medication has become lengthy and complicated. If all goes well, have one more shot to give tomorrow night in this series. Yesterday, the one I gave was too low in belly and it hurt. Tonight, recognizing my previous mistakes and those of nurses at hospital, gave shot which she didn't even feel. When I told her it was over, she thought I was kidding.

She had a good day today, out of bedroom all day with very little pain or nausea. Much more alert and feeling much better. Am beginning to think that if you are sick, hospitals are not the place to get well. It's remarkable the improvement since release. Also, am feeding her smaller meals six times a day. Seems to work better and keeps up the appetite. After getting up and putting medication together, which is a seven-times-a-day chore, prepared breakfast, took temperature, pulse and blood-pressure. Tried to read paper which I finally finished late in the afternoon. Started laundry after breakfast and did four loads. Sister-in-law came in late in morning, so I went to grocery while she was here. She made some cheese spread while I was gone. Michele had arrived so I gave her a birthday card and her gifts. Guess she was pleased. Both stayed about an hour,

Dan stopped by later and then went home to heat up grill to cook steaks promised Michele for her birthday today. Fixed sweet potatoes, hominy and fruit Jello for supper. Then sixth and final snack for day was Fritos and chocolate ice cream. Have been taking temperature four times a day, the final time at 9 p.m. Also final medication for day.

The X-ray was checked again. Instead of tumor greatly enlarged, the new report was a dramatic reduction. So additional MRI and lumbar tap which I had mentioned before were both not necessary but charges of about $1500 remained. Whoever read the wrong X-ray or was careless should be held responsible for causing all that expense, not to mention the pain of going through the tests. Looking back at this day, can't believe that except for reading the newspaper a few minutes at a time, have not stopped the entire blessed day.

May 27, 1996

Have finished supper, medication, temperature, pulse, blood pressure and injection. Can now stop for a moment until bedtime.

Believe that shot tonight of Neupogen is last one, but will have to wait until nurse comes and takes blood tomorrow morning and get results. If white counts are back up, this should be the last one for this time around. More storms coming in tonight. Tried to mow before noon but grass was so wet that it just balled up inside mower so gave up.

I am not giving a speech this year for Memorial Day for the first time in many years. To tell the truth, it almost feels like a relief not to have to go anywhere. But then, perhaps the situation has something to do with that. Today, anybody would be hungry if they stayed in this house for a few minutes from the smell of cooking. I suggested to the doctor that instead of Meryl trying to get down three regular meals a day, we would try six smaller meals. The response was that was a good idea and it's really working. What I didn't anticipate is that her appetite is growing and the small meals and snacks are growing too. Lousy Memorial Day for a day of remembrance although it's used for recreation and picnicking. So rain fell on a day when we ought to be remembering those who went and never came back or are gone now. Perhaps some people will reflect on that, but my guess is that most are fretting about the weather and the loss of a day of recreation.

May 28, 1996

Had to get up early, about 6 a.m., put out trash, put medication together. Then I took temperature, blood pressure and pulse. That was the first of four times which I do everyday. Breakfast was oats, juice, toast and green tea. About 8:45, company that was supposed to install air conditioning and have twice delayed the process showed up. The young man's effort's was worth my change of heart in allowing the company to go ahead with the project. Am going to write a letter as I have never seen a more dedicated and organized person. He constantly cleaned up as he worked, took his shoes off whenever he had to come into the house and was just outstanding. We are having central air installed in order to keep my wife more comfortable during hot weather. The house is large and normally has remained cool over the years, but circumstances are different now.

Nurses came this morning but had no instructions on what to do. Did not even bring proper equipment. They had installed a Metaport in her chest at the hospital so it would not be necessary to pierce into a vein each time an IV was needed or blood taken. Nurse said she would be coming on Monday, Wednesday and Friday of each week. A therapist is to come in a couple times a week. Effects of last chemo are now wearing off and can't believe spouse's appetite. I keep piling more and more on the plate, and it comes back empty. Gave last Neupogen shot last night and nurses were supposed to tell me if more needed. Neither the nurses nor the clinic called back as promised so on my own, decided not to give another shot.

I now am convinced the medical profession is one of the poorest communicators in our society. Wish now I had kept better track of just how many things have been left hanging.

May 29, 1996

Helper showed up this afternoon and I was able to start some mowing. Mower broke after about five minutes and very little done. Worse, because of problem, belt was nicked and had to be replaced. Mowing will have to wait until tomorrow, although helper did get trimming done so mowing ought to be a little easier.

Meryl is getting noticeably better. Last night, in the absence of instructions, decided against giving her a Neupogen injection. Glad I made that decision. I stopped at lab today and picked up copy of blood results, which showed white blood cell count was up to four times normal. If I had given her the shot, hate to think of how much higher it might have gone. Nurse finally called me late this afternoon to tell me to stop. Told her I had already decided to stop. Have started adding more detail to daily notes I have been making. Am beginning to realize this record might be a great help to others who may have to go through this same terrible experience.

May 30, 1996

Nurse was in this morning and took blood. Picked up lab report in afternoon and more improvement. White blood cells, which had sky rocketed to over 40,000, were down to 15. Normal is 10 to 15. Platelets are now in normal range again but red blood cells still are not. But all is improving. Was outside very little today. Decided to do mostly book work today. Got a lot done. Went to Krogers to copy some papers, then groceries and would you know that I forgot folder in cart. Went back to see if anybody had turned it in and no luck. When I got home, telephoned and learned it had been turned it. That was a relief because I had vouchers for two airline tickets and important medical records in the folder. I called the airline today to see if anything could be salvaged if the tickets were not used. The lady with whom I chatted talked to her boss and they agreed to send me two vouchers in the amount paid for the certificates less a $50 deduction on my ticket. Thought that was fair but now have to send them the certificates, a letter of explanation along with the doctor's statement. All that was in the folder as I needed to make copies for my files.

I have been asked to go to Washington on June 12 to brief the Secretary of Defense on job opportunities for service-persons leaving the military in the reduction in defense appropriations. This will entail some preparation but whether I will be able to go depends on health situation. Supposedly, I will be able to return the next day or June 13. As mentioned, health situation is a major consideration as well as the time and research needed to do this properly.

Have to go to Wright-Pat next week. Doctor has given me a bunch of prescriptions that I can have filled. My estimate is that the retail cost is over $1,000.

Therapist was in today. Stayed briefly and left me the responsibility for Meryl's exercise. It was same way at hospital except for the first day. People act concerned and are personable but there is little or no follow-up. Picked up the video, "Bridges of Madison County" tonight. Meryl seems to be up to watching it, I hope.

* * *

DAILY RECORD V

May 31, 1996

Got a lot done today and am trying to think of what all I did. Went out this afternoon and finished repairing the mower. Then back in the house to fill out some forms and write checks that are due. After I had lunch, the lawn helper showed up and had to stop to show him what to do. This right in the middle of temperature, pulse, blood pressure, plus three phone calls all at the same time.

Well, got it all done without putting anybody or anything in jeopardy. While preparing fourth meal of the day, Michele came in and announced she was cooking dinner. The menu was liver, (without onions for me), mashed potatoes, red beets and cake for desert. Sister-in-law arrived after we had started eating and brought a box of Salmon filets. Will broil a couple of those tomorrow night.

Then phone rang and lady with whom I talked last night wanted to look at vacant apartment. She wanted to rent it, so now I have to finish some minor touch up which should take perhaps four or five hours. Got everything mowed with tractor today, except had to go over some places two or three times.

I'm getting a little more caught up. To end the day, took a shower and put wife to bed. I have to wonder how many people who find themselves in this situation are able to cope. Being retired is of course a great advantage except that I have continuing responsibilities. If someone is working full time, that would be most difficult.

June 1, 1996

Have been able to reduce Meryl's pain medicine, although at times pain in legs requires a little Roxanol in juice at bedtime. This seems to allow her to sleep without interruption through the night. She is becoming more mobile -that is, moving around by herself with the aid of a walker. She likes using a dining room chair which is on casters. It is much easier to use than the walker, although not too good on carpet.

Have been taking her outside when weather is okay so she can lie in the sun. However, she has to stop after about a half hour as she seems to become too warm.

Did not get out much today. Went to post office and to grocery store. Otherwise, spent the day cleaning, doing five loads of laundry and cooking. Breakfast was pancake and bacon, lunch was grilled cheese sandwich. Dinner was liver and onions, mashed potatoes and fruit Jello.

Meryl is now in bed and am somewhat tired tonight. It's warm upstairs but just right downstairs so can't turn on air conditioning as it would be too cold downstairs in her room.

June 2, 1996

Have appointment with oncologist Tuesday afternoon. However, if he wants to start another round of chemo, we have agreed to say NO at this time until her physical condition becomes a great deal better than it is at the moment. While the recovery from the last one is obvious, she still has much more to go before another round. I know it's a risk but I think that to go ahead is an even greater risk. Blood still not up to par even though she is feeling better.

This was a most confining day. Intended to go to church this morning but got up later than I had planned and then found events did not allow me to get away. In fact, was out of the house only once all day and that was late this evening to say good-bye to Michele as she was leaving. She came over about 5:30 to help out with supper. Weather is back to furnace time. Rained most of the night and morning and windy rest of day. Am convinced that weather makes a difference in attitudes of people. Spent most of day being nurse and cook.

Little time to myself. Even with Michele's help, still stayed busy. Have some shopping to do but don't know when I will get to it. Michele will be in Toledo until Tuesday. She is going to stay here Wednesday evening so I can go to Governor Rhodes' dinner for former cabinet members. It is in Plain City, about an hour's drive from here. Then Thursday, she is staying again as I have a dental appointment at 1 p.m. That leaves Friday to get to Wright-Pat.

It got dark early here which added to a most unsatisfactory day. Bad weather seems to replace hope with despair. The reduced light and gloomy outdoors reminds me of the night scene in the film, "Fantasia".

Too bad we can't always experience the exhilaration that comes with the new light.

June 3, 1996

We have had tremendous thunder and lightning for the past four hours. There is a small lull right now. One of the tenants had a drain that was sluggish. Was able to get out for a little while this afternoon, pick up mail, go to grocery and take a drain rooter down to apartment. Took about 15 minutes to clear the drain and I was sweating like the can of an ice cold beer on a humid day in July.

Came back home, got a little book work done, then fixed a most simple supper of tomato soup with milk and butter. Later she had some ice cream pie which Michele had made last night.

Am now in my pajamas and getting rather sleepy although I don't know why. Have appointment with oncologist tomorrow morning at 11 a.m. Wife has not yet recovered sufficiently from the last round. Platelets are now in the middle of normal range. White blood count had gone way up after dropping to very low but has now come back down to 50% too high. Red blood count is still much too low and don't think her system could take another round of poisoning right now. Also, it has only been three weeks since last round, so I feel it's too early.

I believe now that they take them to the brink of death and then bring them back. That's really about it only this time, they almost didn't make it back.

June 4, 1996

Doctor wants to start next round of chemo next Tuesday. However, office told us he was all booked up on Tuesday so had to settle for Wednesday. This time, he wants to give her the chemo intravenously in the hospital. Meryl is not sure that she wants to put off chemo, as we had discussed, because she has developed an unusual trust in doctor. But, the decision will depend on how well she comes along during the next week.

Appointment today at medical facility was supposed to be at 11:15 a.m. Got there at 11:05 and was informed it had been canceled. Problem was that nobody bothered telling us. So, wife had to sit in a wheel chair from 11:05 until 12:40 before the doctor got around to seeing her. That is the longest she has been able to sit up for weeks. All together, she was in the wheel chair from 11:05 until 1:30. Doctor said there was nothing he could do about problem. My response was that there was something I could do and I would do it. He told me who to see and said he hoped something would be done to solve lack of coordination.

It seems some people couldn't care less about the suffering they cause just because they don't do their job.

Yard helper is coming, I think, tomorrow afternoon to trim at apartments as well as some other work. Got to keep up now that grass is finally manageable. Don't want it to get out of hand again.

Just got a signal from wife downstairs for some attention. Michele had been in Toledo for a meeting and stopped by on her way home. This is the latest wife has gone to bed in several weeks. Tomorrow is Susan's birthday so will have to find time to get her a card. Guess Michele has taken care of the gift. Medication is all taken now for night, temperature taken, etc. Have been wondering how patients survive without someone to take care of so much detail. I am positive that when something like this happens in many families, the patient does not get all the treatment necessary. Couldn't believe I had to tell the doctor today the dates of the past two chemos, how many days of treatment and what kind. Records I have kept on temperature, blood pressure and pulse that I took with me were not given a second glance. If I hadn't taken a copy of the last blood work, they were going to have her do it again. Nobody had bothered to send a copy to the hospital.

Just got a letter from supplementary insurance. Now they want prior approval on drugs. It is a sign of the times that people make things more difficult.

June 5, 1996

Governor Rhodes' dinner was over earlier than I expected. I sort of anticipated a roast but nothing was really organized, except that a lot of old friends got together. Only speaker was Rhodes. Each time he finished, he thought of something else so that he told one story after another for over forty five minutes.

But I think everyone had a good time. Saw many old friends whom I was glad to see again and who seemed to be glad to see me. Some whom I had expected to see are no longer with us. I sat between

Martin Janus who was in charge of the Department for Aging, and Fred Neunschwander who was development director during Rhodes early years as governor. Thought to take my video camera and many people asked for a copy. So, it looks like another project which I will turn over to Phil Hamilton, who has his own firm but was director of the Department of Administration.

Gov. Rhodes is now in a wheel chair. His knees are causing the trouble. He was barely able to get out of the wheel chair to use walker to take about four steps to car. He said in four years, he will be 90. He wants whoever is left to help him celebrate at another dinner for his old cabinet.

Today was pretty much routine as far as patient is concerned. Day consists of taking temperature at 8 a.m., medication 30 minutes before breakfast, then breakfast with more medication along with special drops in juice. Breakfast was pancakes, syrup, bacon, prune juice and tea. Usually there is a snack in mid morning, but breakfast was so late we went on to lunch. Medication, then pimento cheese sandwich, black corn chips & orange juice. Afternoon snack was pretzels and strawberry milkshake.

Michele arrived about 4:30. I had medication for supper and bedtime all out before I left for the dinner. Main course for dinner at home was stir fried veggies. Snack before bedtime was freezer pie that Michele had made. Ran out of one of the drugs which I was going to pick up at Wright-Pat Friday so had to fill it here.

Tomorrow at 1 p.m., I have a dental appointment. Michele is coming over about noon so I can keep it. Also, she is coming over Friday so I can go to Wright-Pat for more prescriptions.

Canceled my Washington briefing today as Meryl is going into hospital on the same day. But have agreed to put briefing in writing and mail it.

June 6, 1996

Wife's vital signs are now staying fairly close to normal - pulse, blood pressure and temperature. This day started out with oats, toast, Horse Tail Tea or Te de Cola de Coballo (obviously in Spanish) and orange juice.

Michele fixed lunch so I don't know what all that was. After breakfast, snack was pretzels and strawberry milkshake. Supper was tomato soup, tuna salad sandwich, crackers, grape juice and brick cheese. After supper snack was chocolate ice cream and Fritos. Michele stayed with Meryl during my dental appointment.

I was in the dental chair, flat on my back for over 3 hours. Between the student dentist and the female faculty dentist, they managed to make a small job into a big one. They didn't even get the tooth filling finished so now have to go back in a week. I think that a good dentist would have completed the job in less than 45 minutes. But, the young man worked long and carefully although I think he was getting more tired than I was. Went to Wright- Pat today to pick up prescriptions. Was there by 10:30.

We are having many more cloudy days than sunny. What worries me is that when this stops, we may start experiencing no rain and a lot of heat. That would be about all we need. So will think in a more positive manner which means that I will wish for the best and suspect the worst.

June 7, 1996

Temperature, blood pressure and pulse pretty much normal for day. Just finished taking last temperature for day, blood pressure and pulse. Also put together last round of medication.

Meryl has been in bed for almost 45 minutes and is pretty tired. So my guess is that sleep has taken over for this day. Last snack for tonight was chocolate ice cream with Fritos. As much food as is being consumed, would think that she should be weighing a ton by now. Weight is coming back but very slowly. It was lost over a period of more than three months, so it will probably take even longer to get it back. A lot of weight is loss of muscle mass in legs. The only way that can come back is with exercise.

Checked out prescriptions after returning from Wright-Pat and all is correct. Was completely out of two items. Now if I can just get the doctor to continue to give me these prescriptions a couple of weeks in advance, it will makes the trip worthwhile. Had I purchased in local pharmacy, my cost would have been over $1000. This is the first time I have been able to get prescriptions in advance.

June 8, 1996

Was able to get to the garage and have new tires put on Meryl's car, plus lube and oil change. Chef Jim prepared pancakes, bacon, prune juice and tea for breakfast. Had to walk home, then back to garage, a total of about 1 ½ miles. Took care of medication and snack of Ensure. . They finished at 11:50 in time for me to get to bank before noon.

Lunch was pimento cheese, crackers and I forget what else. Snack was another lapse in memory. Supper was grilled ham and cheese sandwich, cottage cheese, pineapple and Jello: Final snack was Three Musketeers bar. Her appetite has come back with a vengeance. Final medication at bedtime and another day has come to an end. Did get paper done about an hour ago for briefing I will not be attending in Washington. Now have to get it to them in time.

June 9, 1996

Can't believe how this day turned out. And the day has not been without its challenges and opportunities. Didn't sleep too well last night. Got up about 6:30. Took temperature which was normal and I left pills to be taken a little later, as I wanted to go to Mass. Got there a few minutes late and left a few minutes early so that I was home by 9 a.m. Breakfast was toast, juice, tea and hot oatmeal. Later, snack was a chocolate milkshake and a couple of wafers.

Meantime, got to read the paper which is huge on Sunday. Lunch was easy - pimento cheese on Ritz crackers and some juice and Jello. Snack was another milk shake. Decided to try mowing. It felt like it was going to rain as a few drops came down but sun came out. Started mowing at 2:30 p.m. and finished a little after 4:30. Had company most of the day, but I still had to get work done. Had already done laundry in morning. Read the briefing I would have given on Wednesday, found some typos, corrected and reprinted. Finally, it was time to get supper together so asked if menu of broiled pork chops, mashed potatoes and cottage cheese with pineapple had any merit. Got agreement on that.

Prepared supper and gave her much more than I thought she would eat. When I went back from kitchen to check if she needed anything else, plate was wiped clean. Final snack was chocolate ice cream. So now, she is in bed. Forgot to take one temperature reading but it didn't make any difference. Temperature is staying fairly steady at 98.6. At times in late afternoon, it might go up a tenth or so, but am amazed at how things have leveled off.

I remember it was like this before last chemo began and then all hell broke loose. Pain, nausea, weakness and totally bed ridden in hospital for twelve days. It was after the release from the hospital that improvement began and progressed rather rapidly. Anyway, it's now just 9 p.m. and its been a long day. Can't believe how much I was able to do. Guess I should understand why I'm feeling a little tired.

June 11, 1996

Red blood count still a little low so started patient on some iron, 400mcg. Probably should be a lot more. Also, added calcium, magnesium and potassium as they are all below normal. As Dr. Narvaez from Juarez would say, not clinically significant. Will continue extra supplements.

Tomorrow we go to the treatment annex. Appointment at 9:40 for first treatment of chemo intravenously, then to hospital where she will get second and third treatments Thursday and Friday. Only three this time with dosage reduced and medicine changed in part. Lab work and chest x-ray will be completed in the morning. Doctor wants first treatment in annex so he can make sure it goes exactly as he wants. Now, Meryl is getting ready for bed and will ring when ready.

The Briefing for Washington got to destination on time. Was told that by 1 p.m. it had been faxed all over the country, including California, and that twenty copies had been made to take with the delegation.

Regretted that I couldn't go, but what I did was the next best and only thing I could do.

Back to daily diary, blood pressure and pulse improving each day and temperature is staying pretty much normal. She picks up a tenth or two in evening but most of the time, it's 98.6. Each day, she seems to be getting stronger and pulse also seems to be getting stronger.

Menu for today was scrambled eggs, sausage, prune juice and toast for breakfast, 2 Snickers Bars for snack, Tuna salad sandwich, cheese and fruit for lunch, freezer pie for snack, stir fried veggies, brown rice, cottage cheese salad for supper and final snack was diet 7-Up and popcorn.

June 12, 1996

I spent most of the day in the hospital and annex. Got up early, started medication at 7 a.m., fixed breakfast of bacon, pancake, juice and tea, then got ready to leave for the clinic. She packed up a few things to take to the hospital and by 9:10 a.m., we were on the way. Doctor wanted to start first round of chemo there so he could personally handle it. However, it was over two hours before he was able to see her.

After short visit, decided to send her to hospital to start chemo as they could handle it all there. Called hospital and arrangements were made. Finally left clinic about 12:45, with blood taken, plus chest and leg X-rays before leaving.

Got to hospital and Michele thought we ought to have lunch. By that time, it was almost 2 p.m. Then checked into admissions and from there, up to ninth floor.

Found that instead of private room, she had a room mate. With what she has to go through, absolutely not acceptable. Head of floor finally came out and spent next twenty minutes telling us it was all unfortunate, that doctor could not dictate where she would be. When I explained that the information came from hospital, not the doctor, her voice only became louder and it got worse.

At this point, I was seeing red so I shut up and let Michele do the negotiating. Won't go into all the details, but told them if they couldn't do better, we would just take her out of hospital. So, put her in room temporarily and about forty-five minutes later, three guys came in and said they were moving her into her own room. Instead of taking her out of bed, they wheeled the entire bed into the private room. The chemo which was supposed to be done early was not done, although they finally started her on IV. Chemo finally arrived four hours late and did not finish until 7:25 p.m.

Nurse told me they would move time up by two hours Thursday and again Friday. That would, if it works out, get her finished Friday by 3:25 p.m., after which she is supposed to be discharged. But am not holding my breath.

I stayed until nearly 8 p.m. and then came home. After fixing a bite to eat, decided to get this all down before I have forgotten. May have to go to Wright-Pat either tomorrow or Friday, depending on which day works out. Have another batch of prescriptions to pick up and these are really expensive.

June 13, 1996

Meryl is still in hospital, but is supposed to be released tomorrow. Also, will get last chemo treatment for this round after which she will be released. Have prescriptions for treatment after the chemo is done so decided go to Wright-Pat today as that seemed to fit the schedule best.

Got up early this morning, left for hospital about 9 a.m., everything seemed okay there so took off for the base. Arrived there about 11 a.m., was almost an hour and half getting prescriptions filled. Turned out they were out of one prescription so will have to pick it up locally. Even so, total of prescriptions, had I bought them locally, came to over $4,000. Next, stopped at commissary to pick up a few items and was back home by 3 p.m. Put medication in refrigerator as it must be kept between 36 and 56 degrees, picked up mail and then left for hospital. Stayed until about 8:30 p.m. when chemo was finished.

Last round will take about an hour and wife is supposed to be released tomorrow. This morning, before I left hospital, 1 checked to make sure they had moved the time two hours so that it would be given two hours earlier, with another two hours for Friday. Otherwise, It would not be finished on Friday until 7:30 and it would be dark when released.

When I asked at desk, person there said he knew nothing about it and couldn't do anything. Fortunately, the pharmacist was standing there and he said he'd look it up in the medical records. It was not there so he told me that he would personally take care of it. I thanked him for doing what I thought was a most logical thing to do. And he did take care of it, except that the nurse was half hour late getting it started.

But if plan works, she should be finished tomorrow by 3:30 p.m. that is if there isn't another goof.

June 14, 1996

Day went okay. Got up, dressed, and prepared to leave for hospital about 10:00 this morning. Went to post office first and remembered a couple of things I had forgotten. So came back to house,

243

dropped off mail and started out again for the hospital. Got there about 10:45, everything was okay so took off to do a quick errand.

Doctor's assistant gave me three typed pages outlining home instructions. Things went pretty much on schedule and a new nurse, her name was Mary Margaret, with a nickname of Mar- gee pronounced like the "g" in glee. She got all the IV's going with the last being the chemo. Even though she was off at 3 p.m., she stayed until nearly 4 to make sure that the process didn't get delayed with another nurse. In fact, for the last hour she was there, other than typing up some stuff for her computer, she spent all her time getting everything ready so that there would be no delay in the discharge.

Am absolutely amazed at the contrast in the way people react to such situations. Seems as though it's either feast or famine. There's no in between.

Got home about 4:30 p.m. and back into routine. Supper was ham, cottage cheese salad and hominy. Gave spouse a pretty large amount of food and the plate was cleaned. But then came a real surprise. For the first time in months, she walked without support a couple of times back and forth in the living room. I was amazed as her legs are so weak. Bed time came about 8:45 p.m. and legs ached a little. There is a salve we brought back from Juarez which helps reduce pain.

A tired patient didn't take long to get to sleep. Using salve, hot towels and heating pads on her legs has been an almost nightly routine since about the first day of our arrival in Juarez. While I have not had to do this every night, there are nights when her legs are so painful that this seems to be the only relief. However, the pain has been easing off and the need for heat and pads is also reduced. In the meantime, Neupogen shots start again tomorrow for ten days.

June 15, 1996

After breakfast this morning, Dan and I were going to a computer sale near Westerville. Dan called about 9 a.m. and said he couldn't go as Susan had a hair appointment. He had to stay with boys. I went alone and when I got there, must have been two hundred or more people waiting in line. My first impulse was to leave. Then I realized that the place had not opened yet. They opened doors just as I got there. Took about three minutes to get in. Looked around, found some odds and ends, then it took almost forty-five minutes to pay for purchases.

Came back to Gahanna, stopped at post office, then home. Snack had already been eaten so other than medication and lunch, that was it. Took ham out of freezer to thaw and later baked. Perhaps this is the best one yet. Tasted it about 5:30 and it was delicious, even if I do say so. But back to after lunch, opened mail and found bills for twelve-day hospital stay of over $25,000. All together, the bills totaled over $30,000 counting other charges. Then on the bottom, it stated, "This is not a bill".

June 16, 1996

Got up about 6:30 a.m., took care of preliminaries and first medication, then went to Mass. Fixed breakfast when I returned, had time to read paper and morning was nearly over. Dan stopped by with Fathers' Day card which was one pun after another. He stayed a couple of hours.

Michele and Dan gave me a pair of walking sneakers but of course, they didn't fit. So went out following lunch, after Dan had left and Michele had arrived. Tried on about two dozen pairs of shoes and finally took a pair I didn't like, but nothing else fit. Got back about 4:30 p.m. and decided to try to mow since Michele was going to fix dinner. Got about half done and will try to finish tomorrow.

Meantime, the dinner Michele fixed involved heating up some food a neighbor had brought in yesterday. It was a young lady with whom I had served on a committee once who heard about the illness. She brought in five bags of food including lasagna, roast beef pot roast, barbecue beef, stick rolls, buns, and chips, just to mention a few of the items. I was absolutely amazed. Will have to show my appreciation somehow. Started the first of ten Neupogen shots yesterday. After today, eight more to go for this round.

Also, Monday, will start another shot, Epogen, to be given on Monday, Wednesday and Friday for four weeks, or a total of fourteen shots. This one is supposed to build up red blood count. The Neupogen works on the white blood cells. Have given Neupogen shots after each course of chemo but this is the first time for Epogen.

According to the explanation that came with the drug, it is supposed to reduce the need for transfusions. Also, a nurse will be coming three times a week starting tomorrow to take blood. Meryl went outside this morning for about a half hour and sat in sun. At end of time, she was perspiring and became dizzy. Took a cool, wet towel and dried

245

her off. After short rest, was okay again and she came inside. Was afraid too much exposure would cause sunburn, which could cause a great deal of trouble. But all is well. As usual after mowing, am sneezing so took an Echinacea capsule. Will finish mowing tomorrow.

While pain medication has been cut back, at times the pain comes back in her legs. I have to give her some Roxonal, a narcotic pain reliever with some juice. Also, I think that I now have made the sixth revision to the medication schedule.

* * *

DAILY RECORD VI

June 17, 1996

Another long day with little time to relax. Up at 5:30 a.m., took out trash, then medication. Breakfast was pancakes, bacon (delicious), grape juice, prune juice, tea, then orange juice. Afterward, spouse went outside for a half hour. This is two days in a row she has done this. Yesterday, she got overheated and was dizzy when she got up. Put her in the shade to cool off. No problem today, but sun wasn't as hot. Snack was Ensure and pretzels. Medication, then lunch, post medication after hot dog, veggies, fruit Jello. Medication is seven times a day, both pre and post food. Some medication is taken thirty minutes before eating and the rest after. So with breakfast, lunch and dinner, that makes six times with one more at bedtime.

She is no longer taking morphine except for a mild pill at bedtime. Don't think she really needs that but nurse thought it would be better to taper off gradually. So that is down from four times a day to just the one. Snack in afternoon was tuna, cheese and crackers.

My yard helper showed up, so I was able to finish the mowing I started yesterday. It took about an hour and a half. Helper did the trimming and we finished shortly before it started raining. Michele stopped by twice with supplies.

With final taking of temperature for day, another day of many days is coming to an end. Still take temperature four times a day, also blood pressure and pulse. Temperature has been pretty much normal but blood pressure and pulse vary a great deal. Also today, started the Epogen shot which is in addition to the Neupogen shot. The Epogen is a new one that stimulates red blood cells and platelets. Neupogen is every day with seven more to go.

June 18, 1996

Television news announced that nearly two inches of rain fell in the Columbus area in a very short time this evening. Rain drops have been huge. In just ten minutes or so, everything was literally flooded.

Gave fourth Neupogen shot tonight with some apprehension. White blood count was double normal yesterday but didn't feel that I should stop yet. They did that at hospital and started again too late. Tomorrow, will give the second Epogen shot along with Neupogen if white blood count is not too high. Doctor says not to worry but instructions say otherwise.

Meryl has a healthy appetite. Ham, eggs, prune juice, grape juice, toast, tea for breakfast. Snack was tuna, cheese and crackers. Lunch was Jello and pimento cheese sandwich, with another snack of a chocolate milkshake. Dinner was French fries and a huge fish sandwich, of which hardly anything was left. Final snack was Jello and wafers.

Critical time is approaching from last chemo and legs were aching tonight. Worse time will be from Friday to Monday. This is the time that there will be a possible need for transfusion of whole blood and/ or platelets. Am hoping that Epogen will eliminate that. However, according to data that came with drug, it will be four to five weeks before it starts taking effect. Nurse is due to take blood tomorrow morning.

Right now, weather is calm, no rain, thunder or lightning. Television report says more possible until 11 o'clock. Tomorrow is supposed to be a nice day. House is staying very comfortable so hot weather has not been a problem so far.

June 19, 1996

Seems that things kind of get into a rut and days become very much like each other. Got up about 6:50 a.m., shaved, then went down, had a banana, juice, vitamins, but can't for the life of me remember what else. Wake up time today was 7:30 a.m. as nurse was to be here by 9:30 a.m. Breakfast was oats, the real kind fixed the old way, juice, tea, pills, and toast. Nurse could not get blood from either port. This surgical invention doesn't work most of the time, another nurse has told me. It's greatest attribute appears to be the cost for the operating room and the surgeon's fee. It will accept stuff going in but stops up when blood is withdrawn. Sort of acts like a check valve. Nurse injected a bunch of

248

anti- coagulant into both ports and took blood from the arm. Modern medicine - still barbaric and crude.

Am working a little each day now on taxes and hope to get them done sometime in next couple of weeks or so. But days are long with constant need to do things. I doubt that I have more than a couple of free hours each day. Am beginning to realize why I am a little tired when the time comes to retire. I went to the library early in the week and picked up seven books on cancer. I am curious and must learn more.

June 20, 1996

Was thinking on the way to the post office today about how to recognize art. It is art if one sees something and has to guess what it is. Dan just called me to ask about a stock that some broker called him about. He was telling about an article in the Wall Street Journal about how someone threw darts at the stock listings and made out better than the Standard and Poors Index. Told him that I had also read it and that it was really a sticky point. His groan could be heard without a telephone. Need a little humor through all this.

Bedtime is getting a little later. So far, this round of chemo seems to be a little better but am keeping fingers crossed. For daily menu, breakfast-eggs, link sausage, prune juice, tea and toast with apple butter. Snack was root beer with Frittos, Lunch-tuna sandwich, cheese and Jello. Snack was Ensure and wheat thins. Dinner was a hot ham sandwich, hominy and Jello. Snack was spumoni ice cream and Frittos. Sounds like a lot, but eaten at a rate of six times per day, guess it goes down easily.

I'm beginning to see a filling out of loose skin, so my belief is that she is gaining weight. Scales show only about five pounds from a low of 106 but she looks heavier. Gave another Neupogen shot tonight. Am getting quite good at it. No pain and no blood.

Think I'll start injecting myself, Ha.

Am very low on two medications. Michele was in Boston today. Dan has depositions, among other things, so no chance to get to Wright-Pat. Not really worth the trip for just two items anyway, so will pick them up locally. These are not expensive. Just got called and wife now bedded down for night.

Went out for a few minutes this afternoon, and cut poison ivy and oak vines that were climbing trees. Checked apricot tree and there

249

are several apricots still there. Animals are taking them off and dropping them on the ground. Apple trees are loaded, but many on ground also.

June 21, 1996

Was inside most of the day except for this morning. Menu today: Breakfast, pancakes, bacon, juice, tea. Snack-ensure and Frittos. Lunch-grilled cheese sandwich, Jello. Snack-couple of candy bars. Dinner-broiled fish, fried rice and Jello. Final snack- chocolate ice cream. Tonight was double shot, both Neupogen and Epogen.

No more Epogen now until Monday. Seventh Neupogen shot today. Normally, three more to go unless more is needed. Both ports in Metaport did not work because of clots, but one opened up this morning. They put medication in the other to try to open it up but no success.

Woke up about 4:30 a.m. and could not go back to sleep. Finally got up a little after 5 o'clock and got things started. Had to pick up a couple of prescriptions. Later, picked up lab blood report. Both red and white were way down, especially big drop in white. It has gone from four times too high to 50% too low in just four days. Called doctor and reported.

He immediately decided on a transfusion tomorrow morning at 8:30. He had made up an order by the time we finished talking and said the hospital would call and confirm. If they did not call within two hours, I was to call him at home. I waited three hours, then called him. Wife answered and he was out.

The doctor called back about 9 o'clock and said the time was changed to 4:30 p.m. He then said to get there at 3 o'clock because that might speed up the process. I was wondering how I could give the Neupogen shot on time because of the appointment, when the phone rang. It was a woman at the hospital, saying they could not reach me. I said I had not left the house and phone had not rung. Then she told me they had been trying to call the wrong number, although the doctor had given them correct one. I think the doctor was more than a little peeved and stirred things up a little. But she also stated the time had been changed again and now was scheduled for 11:30 a.m. That takes care of my Neupogen shot problem.

It seems that each hierarchy has its special area of authority and nobody, believe me, nobody dares to tread. Doctor told me if he isn't careful, he gets no cooperation from nurses. He asked me to report my feelings to the hospital administrator. Even gave me his name.

Now for my newest cooking accomplishments - fried rice and a fruit Jello, with mandarin orange slices, crushed pineapple, sectioned apricots and walnuts.

June 22, 1996

White and red blood counts all plunged from Wednesday so Meryl is getting a transfusion today. Neupogen has caused pain in hips and legs. Kept her awake a couple of nights now. Last night, insisted that she take some Roxanol which is a break-through pain medicine. Seems to have worked as she was not awake very long.

It's been a long day. Left for hospital about 10:45 a.m. Thought we would be back by about 4:00 o'clock. Finally got back at 8:15 p.m. They gave her two packets of whole blood, other stuff before and after, then checked blood. Everything had come up except platelets had dropped more. Not critical yet. They will take blood again Monday to see if more transfusions are necessary.

Later, went to grocery and picked up items needed, including bottled water. Had to wait at hospital as no wheel chairs available. They finally picked her up and I went to garage to park. Went to area where she was to go and girl at desk did not know where she was. Then she learned Meryl had been taken to a room without the desk being notified. If the late-afternoon appointment had not been changed, we would still have been at the hospital, probably until after midnight.

Only had breakfast to fix which was oats, toast, juice and tea. Snack tonight was ice cream and Frittos. So, have done very little today except that doing nothing all day but being in hospital is not only tiring but also stressful. Nurse was curious about alternative treatment in Mexico but she was also a staunch supporter of conventional treatment. She had no curiosity at all about what kind of treatment was given.

Guess there are two kinds of doctors and nurses in medical profession, those who do nothing but conventional treatment and all the other "quacks" who perhaps have found that unconventional methods have merit.

Many of these non-traditional doctors have been hounded and harassed. I am reading a book written by a doctor describing his encounters with the news media.

Unbelievable how some reporters totally misrepresented the interviews with him. He had the foresight to tape record all interviews and was able to get retractions.

June 23, 1996

Today was a little different. Didn't get up in time to go to church. Took care of usual needs, breakfast was cream roll, juice, tea. Lunch was pimento cheese sandwich and Jello. Dinner was salmon patties, plus macaroni and cheese. Served the usual three snacks in between.

Told Dan and Michele I have to finish renovating the apartment today as new tenant wants to move in this week. So Dan came over about 9:45 a.m.. We divided the work that was left and were finished by 1:30 p.m. He stayed down for another hour and repaired gutters which were loose in places on other buildings. Still have some damage to repair on the outside which I had not noticed before. Tenant can move in now. Place is clear and ready to occupy.

Michele is leaving tomorrow morning for the west coast. She will be in Washington, Oregon and California until next Sunday and back sometime late Sunday night. Dan wants me to go to Zanesville to do a report on a dryer that blew out the glass in a laundromat and injured a lady who was doing her laundry.

Need to go before the end of the week but will have to figure out how to get someone to stay while I am gone. Won't take long to do study but it will require about two hours each way driving time. Have to take along another engineer as it would not look right to have Dan's dad as an expert witness in the trial.

June 24, 1996

Things back to normal today. Blood work taken this morning and all systems have improved. White blood took a dramatic jump and went over the normal high. This was expected. I know it will climb a great deal higher by Wednesday, then will start back down.

Gave what should be the last Neupogen shot tonight (for white blood cells) but will be giving Epogen shots (for red blood cells) Monday, Wednesday and Friday for three more weeks. I am doing a few things on my own because of the needs I detect, based on the lab work.

As a result, I am providing potassium, calcium, and other supplements as blood work shows these are low. Don't think the medical profession has much concern about minerals. Yet, they are part of the results of blood lab work. If they are not important, why bother?

I have heard about DHEA? It seems that this is a very vital material that the body produces but as we get older, we have less and less. By the time we are in our 60's, many have lost over 80% of what we normally should have. DHEA is available by prescription. Wild Mexican Yam will cause the body to begin producing what is needed and is available without prescription. But who knows!

Decided to start mowing again today. Got most of area around house done but then had to leave for a short time. By the time I got back, it was really storming. So, looks like I will be cutting the grass tomorrow. Perhaps it's better to do a little at a time instead of doing it all at once.

Have been looking at schedule. Wife goes to hospital for chest X-ray and cat scan on July 2. I have a radio program on July 3 for about two hours, and the annual parade is July 4.

Riley will be in his BDUs (battle dress uniform) from Ft. Knox and will ride in the Jeep with me. I am not sure if I can get away with that without grandson Nicholas getting upset. Am already accused of showing favoritism. Michele, as I mentioned previously, is on West Coast until Sunday evening. Dan is tied up so no help from that direction. But am now able to be gone for an hour or so at a time, depending upon the time of day.

Temperature, blood pressure and pulse four times a day. Medication seven times a day -three times before meals, three times after meals and once before bed. Also, shots every day for the past ten days including tonight. Have to make up new medication schedule it seems quite often as prescriptions keep changing. Each time, have more drugs left that will not be used.

June 25, 1966

Finally got grass finished today. Did part yesterday, part this morning and finished after lunch. Seems like it took a lot longer that way but then, each part was rather short and not so boring.

Made pimento cheese this afternoon for future sandwiches. Bacon and eggs this morning, grilled cheese sandwich, hominy and Jello for lunch and hot ham, corn and Jello for supper. No shots today as last Neupogen was yesterday. However, an Epogen shot is due tomorrow.

Have had several calls from in and out of state in last few days requesting that I speak at various functions. Turned down all so far including three more today. Hate to do it as it is the one thing I probably enjoy doing as much as anything, but I have no choice. The situation is totally demanding with no let up of any kind except for the Fort Knox meeting. Right now, with Michele out of town, can't see even being able to go to Wright/Pat to pick up prescriptions. Will be out of several in just a few days and will probably have to get locally. So, my story is not the most encouraging but will survive this ordeal, one way or the other.

Was surprised at how cool it was today. Looked like a real hot day outside but had a long sleeve shirt on while mowing. Big problem right now is that poison ivy and oak is worse than I have ever seen it. Will have to buy some kind of weed killer to try to get rid of it. And am having real problems with birds and squirrels plus other animals, I think. Have never seen so many birds and squirrels. They are tearing up trees.

The upshot of all this is that the entire apricot crop is now gone, and the tree was loaded. One apple tree has only a few left and the other has more on the ground than left on the tree. Nature lovers would enjoy watching all the animals playing, but I watch them and realize how much damage they are doing. Good thing we don't depend on the crops.

June 26, 1996

For several days, have not been away for more than 45 minutes at a time except when Michele has been here. Then, the time has been spent catching up on mowing, getting apartments ready, etc. That is, except for the two trips and the speech at Ohio University.

Blood count back from this morning. Everything has improved except platelet count, which dropped again. Nearing danger point, but think will be okay until blood is taken again on Friday. If platelets drop again, then they will want her in hospital for platelet transfusion.

Gave a Epogen shot tonight and am hoping that the medication begins to take affect. From the start, the information that came with the drug states that it is usually two to six weeks before any significant change occurs. This is only the second week. I still do not understand why this was not started sooner. Some pain has returned in wife's legs, mostly about bed time. I have been giving her some pain breakthrough medication, which takes effect before the regular medication. Has worked for the past three nights. Action comes very quickly and she is getting a good night's sleep as a result.

Breakfast this morning-pancake, ham, prune juice and tea. Snack was crackers and pimento cheese. Lunch was tuna on rye and cheddar cheese slices with fruit Jello. Snack was more crackers. Dinner, beef wieners and my special fried potatoes. Last snack was chocolate ice cream and marshmallows. Weight is coming back, with 10 new pounds added according to scales here at home.

Dan stopped by tonight for a couple of hours. Later, Susan came with both boys and stayed perhaps a half hour. They all left about an hour ago. All quiet now, except for computer keys clicking.

June 29, 1996

Got home about 9:50 a.m. from speech and sister-in-law was ready to leave. No problems while I was gone. She had an appointment, but seemed to know that I wouldn't let her down. She was gone by 10 a.m. which was her deadline. Dan and Susan are having a party for Nicholas tomorrow afternoon. Think I'll go to church in the morning and Meryl wants to go to Dan's tomorrow. Should not be a problem, since I take her back and forth from both the hospital and the clinic. This would be a much shorter ride, and much less effort going and coming. Then later in day, if things go well, will go down to apartment and put on new door hardware. Bought new locks last week and it will take about fifteen minutes to take off old and put on new.

June 30, 1996

Left for Dan's this morning and Meryl used a cane to get around. This was the first time that has happened. She did not even use a walker, which surprised everyone. Thought we would only be there perhaps ten minutes but ended up staying more than two hours.

She had shrimp, salad and hamburger. Dan cooked hamburgers, Brats, hot dogs and barbecued chicken. However, we left before the rest was finished. Meryl didn't want to be there when invited guests arrived.

Took her temperature when we got back and it was up about a half degree. Dropped by bedtime, but this is the problem with being exposed. Couldn't believe Riley. First youngster I ever saw who likes shrimp. By the time his mother cut him off, he had eaten eight huge shrimp and was raring for more. No sauce or anything. Then, when they fixed him a hamburger, he pointed out there was no cheese. Next, he took about two bites and was full.

This has been a hot, humid day here. Air conditioner has been running more than it has been off. There is a stream of water coming out of the unit that looks like an open faucet. But house has been very comfortable. I hate to think of Meryl's discomfort if it hadn't been installed.

July 1, 1996

Blood tests reduced to once a week for now. Got back results this afternoon and everything is improving except red blood count. After each round of chemo, it is harder and takes longer to recover.

Am getting worried that liver and kidneys are being damaged. Dan, Michele and I have decided that if lab work does not show her condition to be in tip top shape by the time next chemo is to start, we are going to hold off until system recovers. Did not need platelets transfusion this time but came very close. Perhaps Epogen is the reason.

Spent part of afternoon working more on taxes. Deadline is August 15 and am beginning to wonder if I will be able to finish by then. Problem is I am only able to work about and hour or two each day. Tomorrow morning, have to go to hospital for X-ray and cat scan. Then I will try to mow in afternoon, also want to replace door locks on apartment that new tenant moved into this past weekend. Helper called today and says he is coming tomorrow. It's more than two weeks late. He said his doctor would not let him work.

July 2, 1996

No food or no drink for patient this morning for two hours prior to X-ray and cat scan, so breakfast was at 7:15 a.m. We were off to the hospital by 8:55 a.m. Things went like clockwork for a change and we were home by 10:35 a.m.

Do not know results yet. After lunch, made a couple of phone calls, worked on taxes for about an hour, then out to mow. Stopped for awhile when Michele showed up with her college roommate from Detroit with whom she has remained close friends.

Spouse had slight temperature at supper time, but okay at bedtime. After mowing and dinner, I went to library and checked out six books on tape. Wife spends a great deal of time listening. Difficult for her to make out printed books, since drugs seem to have impaired her vision. Meryl had vision problems from medication early on in her illness. She enjoys the recorded books, however. May be better than reading once you get used to it.

Returning from the library, I stopped at new tenant's apartment and installed two new door locks. Keys have been lost for back door and front door lock is about worn out.

Got back home about 7:40 p.m. in time for evening snack of chocolate ice cream and mini-marshmallows. And so another day has come to an end. A little surprised at how much I was able to get done.

July 3, 1996

After completing morning care-giver duties, took off for radio station for scheduled interview. Program was from 1:30 to 2:30 p.m., but I stayed an extra half hour to answer an unbelievable number of phone calls from listeners.

Two women who called both said the program was too short and they would have called during the program but didn't want to interrupt. Finally left a little after 3 p.m. The man who did the interview was a World War II veteran and had served in the Army Air Corps. He was one of the few who had flown a B32 bomber. Only eight were built and none survived.

Wife is now in bed. Riley is excited about being in the parade tomorrow morning.

July 4, 1996

It does not seem possible that everything which occurred today actually happened. Riley called me three times this morning prior to the parade. Never saw anyone so excited. A World War II Jeep with two former sergeants, both of World War II vintage, showed up on driveway at exactly 10 a.m.

Dan and Susan had not yet arrived at our house with Riley, so I told them to go on to parade assembly point and we would catch up. Just after they left, Dan showed up. Riley was in his BDU's (Battle dress uniform) from Ft. Knox with a helmet. He had forgotten his sun glasses so I found him a pair. We went to the parade grounds and caught up with the Jeep, although we had to wait about thirty minutes for the parade to start.

When it was our turn to move out, the driver could not get the Jeep started. We lost our place among the politicians while we worked on the Jeep. Finally got it started but then had to wait until all politicians had moved out. They put us directly in front of the band which turned out to be the best place to be. Riley was fascinated with the band behind us, and he was absolutely a model the entire parade.

When we reached our driveway, I had forgotten he wanted some candy to throw out to the crowd along the streets. Michele was waiting with a bag for him. He doled out the candy very carefully the rest of the way, making sure he had some left for himself. At four years old, he acted quite mature and as I introduced him to a number of people, he shook hands with all of them.

End of parade was jammed and we could not get out of parking lot. Did not get home until almost 1 p.m Susan wanted him to change to shorts, but could not get him out of BDU's. Just heard a bang so fireworks have started here in Gahanna. Can see them out of window in upstairs room. Dan got videos of parade and Michele got a couple of pictures, I think. Wife was wheeled out so she could see at least part of the parade, but she stayed out for the whole thing.

Newspaper photographer took picture of Riley so expect to see it in paper soon. Everyone left about 2 p.m. as Dan's neighbors were having a block party at end of their road. One of his neighbors bought over $400 in fireworks so it ought to be a real blast. Except for breakfast which was bananas, oatmeal, juice, tea and toast, did no cooking today.

Perfect day for parade. Skies were clear, weather was dry and temperature was just about right. A lot of older men, and women, saluted as we went by. Nice gesture and I appreciated it. So, here we are, now about 9:45 p.m. and another Independence Day will soon be in the memory books.

Meryl had a pretty good day and I think that perhaps it was her most enjoyable day since cancer diagnosis.

* * *

DAILY RECORD VII

July 5, 1996

I am going to Wright-Pat to pick up more medication tomorrow. Dan is coming over and will be relieved by Michele, who will come later in the day. Think they may be planning on taking Meryl to Michele's so she can see the new draperies Michele had installed. This sort of surprised me but then, if she can go to the hospital, guess going to Michele's house about ten minutes from here shouldn't be a problem.

Went outside for a few moments this morning to get something out of garage. When I returned, wife was doing laundry. Hadn't planned on doing it until week-end, but took over to finish.

A journalism student came about 2 p.m. to interview me at the house. Didn't think it would last very long, but he taped the whole thing and took some notes. We spent an hour and a half. He wanted to know if I would consider giving him a little more time, as he had more questions. Told him that was fine with me, and asked that he call to set up a time.

Not certain what time I will be able to leave for Wright-Pat tomorrow, but am guessing between 9-9:30 a.m. Should be back no later than 2 p.m. Will go to pick up prescriptions first, then to commissary. Wife's appetite continues to be a blessing and a source of comfort.

July 6, 1996

Returned from Wright-Pat just after 3 p.m., then got everything unloaded and put away. Michele left about a half hour after I arrived. Riley is spending the night with her. Got a call from a neighbor informing me that woods next to creek were on fire, and he had called the fire department. Had not been outside since getting home and had no idea anything was happening.

Went outside and sure enough, creek bank next to the driveway from the main street was ablaze. Flames were shooting up about 25 feet. Tried to get out the garden hose, but had so much junk in front that it was impossible. Grabbed a big bucket and started filling and dumping.

After I had done this about a half dozen times, firefighters arrived. They brought a tanker onto the yard and had the fire out in about thirty minutes. Problem now is some rather deep ruts in the lawn where the wheels on the truck sank into the ground. Better than a fire out of control, however. Ironically, I had hired all three of the firemen during my last year as township trustee. The truck was one of two purchased that same year. As they were putting away hoses, another call came in for another fire. Saw the trucks go by including the ladder truck, so it might have been serious. Leaving, the truck went down the driveway to the main street rather than try to back up or turn around.

Wife decided on more spaghetti tonight so made it the same way as the last time. Only change was that the tomato mix which comes in a can has big lumps of tomatoes. I dumped it in the blender before heating it. Wife ate a great supper and I can see improvement each day. I have to remember the doctor warned that cancer could spring up with a vengeance. Also, am concerned that chemotherapy is not as effective as it was the first time. But doctor claims that tumors are getting smaller and wife is happy about that, as am I.

July 8, 1996

Got buzzed just now and had to go down-stairs to prepare some medication. If leg aches are too bothersome, I give her medication in orange juice. It solves the problem very quickly.

Got lab work back this afternoon. Most is considerably better but red blood count and hemoglobin are not showing much improvement. Would indicate that kidneys are not sending proper signal to bone marrow, but both liver and kidney tests do not show a problem. Also, could be a problem with iron. Platelet count, however, did take a huge jump and is now back in normal range. Glad that transfusion was not necessary.

Breakfast was bacon, pancakes, juice and tea. Lunch was barbecue sandwich, plus cottage cheese with onion and green pepper. Broiled a sirloin for supper. with some frozen greens and a salad. Final snack for day was Spumoni ice cream with Munch n' Crunch. She had been asking for some and finally found it at commissary.

Tried some and it tastes like Cracker Jacks. I remember when I used to set up window displays for my Dad in his confectionery when I was about five years old. Could weigh out candy and change a $20 bill.

If that were to happen today, he probably would have been arrested for child cruelty. Am sure glad that I had that early education, but conditions today will not allow that sort of thing. All the busy bodies have managed to make mediocrity the standard. Much of what life demands can no longer be learned during the formative years. Now have to wait until habits have been formed and learning is the exception rather than the rule.

July 9, 1996

Looked at trees this morning and decided that it has become urgent to spray them. But also, leaves are falling as they turn yellow because of a lack of rain. Am not sure just how long it has been since we had rain but I know that it is now perhaps two weeks. Grass is about 50% brown and people are watering like crazy. Not me however. Don't need the extra mowing. New central air conditioning is fine. It might have run a couple of times but the house has stayed cooler than one might have imagined.

Worked on taxes again today. It seems that this year is taking a lot longer than usual, but everything is more complicated and time consuming. Some of the information that goes into the return will end this year so perhaps next year will be easier. But then, come to think about it, the medical expense this year is going to be a chore for next year's return.

Also, there is the matter of closing up the office, which we are trying to do this month, along with the final return for her business. Meryl has done little or no work this year, and doubt very much that she will be able to in the future. She is debating now about renewing her psychologist's license which has risen in cost to $225.

Broiled pork chops tonight, collard greens, with macaroni and cheese on the side. Michele came in just as I finished preparations. Had a feeling that might happen so had put on an extra pork chop. The hunch paid off as she was hungry.

Meryl's appetite continues to bring joy to all of us, and I know her morale is way up.

July 10, 1996

Office has not been closed yet, but gave landlord notice that we intend to do so by early August. Am going to let movers do it all. Don't know exactly what we're going to do with all the furniture and equipment. Dan and Michele are to come over this weekend to try to finalize how this will be done.

Unfortunately, it's another added job which is not needed right now, but cost of maintaining office without anyone there is over $1,000 per month. So, it's time to do something. I don't believe that it will ever be used again. However, we hesitate to make the decision for psychological reasons. Although Meryl suggested it a couple of weeks ago, we still held off to make sure that's what she wanted.

She seems to be having a little pain at night in her legs and takes some extra pain medication at bedtime. Takes effect in an hour or so and then is okay for rest of night.

Have appointment with doctor Monday and am guessing he will want to put her in the hospital again for another round of chemo. If red blood has not really gotten well into normal levels by then, we have agreed that we will decline the next round for the time being.

What good is going through all this if in the process, the liver and kidneys are destroyed. Another serious thought is taking her to Tijuana, Mexico, for some alternative treatment to build her body and strength. If so, will have to get taxes finished and office closed. Treatment is twenty-three days from arrival until finished. Boy, timing is terrible and pressure grows. But, this too shall pass and will feel some relief as the complications are resolved. Wife's condition has not gotten any worse or any better since last round of chemo, at this point.

July 11, 1996

Wife's condition starting to improve. Also, still giving Epogen shots, although not today. Next is tomorrow. Blood taking now down to one day each week. Am still not happy with red counts although platelets are fine. Other counts also are not back to normal.

She is still experiencing pain in legs at bedtime.

July 12, 1996

Two more neighbors called today and said they were tired of waiting for me to call them for help. One lady came over this morning and brought an Amish cake loaf. Delicious. This afternoon, another lady brought chicken salad, croissants and a pineapple upside-down cake. So, chef had a vacation tonight from cooking.

Used last Epogen shot tonight, although don't know why only twelve shots were prescribed. After reading the information that came with the prescription, it appears that once this is started, it's more or less a longer term thing which continues for at least three or four months, or more if needed.

Red blood counts are still low and have actually dropped a little more, although they are not in the danger area. White total blood very normal as are platelets. In reading about all this stuff, it would appear that kidneys and/or bone marrow are not functioning as they should.

Well, next appointment is Monday morning and we will see. Have definitely decided we will not agree to more chemo at this time. Damaging kidneys and liver with chemicals doesn't make sense. Guess the medical profession can say that they took care of the cancer but patient was not able to handle complications. So, Monday morning may be a disagreeable event with doctor, but if she goes into another round of chemo now, it is certain in my mind that kidneys may not recover and several transfusions will be necessary.

In the meantime, body is not getting enough oxygen with low red count. So much for the medical knowledge that I am accumulating. My wife has stated several times she doesn't think she would have survived if I hadn't taken the responsibility to do all the things that I have been doing. It makes me wonder about other cancer patients who must depend entirely on the system. Where is all the progress we keep reading about?

July 13, 1966

The percentage of success with chemotherapy for small cell lung cancer that has spread is less than 5% of survival for two years. Still, they put people through terrible torture, and for what, I'm not sure. As one surgeon stated, he will retire with a most successful career of cutting, but did not contribute one thing toward a cure. At least, there are a few who are honest. The approach is to reduce the tumor but that doesn't cure the cancer. And many will agree that unless the body's immune system goes to work, all the drugs in the world are not going to do any good.

Rained sometime last night. Sprayed fruit trees with bug spray and weeds with weed killer, and wouldn't you know that it would rain right away. I will have to do it again, but will wait until a hurricane approaching Florida is over.

Cooking is becoming a challenge as I look for something new. But tonight, had to make what are in my wife's opinion, my now famous potatoes. Would you believe that no matter how many I make, they disappear as fast as I can make them. So dinner was barbecue sandwich, potatoes, cucumbers and onions. Snack tonight was pineapple upside-down cake with vanilla ice cream. Now all is quiet, wife is in bed and I hope asleep. I'm about to brush my teeth, finish up a couple of things in the office and then go to bed.

July 14, 1996

Had discussion this afternoon with son and daughter. Michele is not in favor of going to Tijuana, because of her concern about Meryl's ability to withstand the long trip. Dan thinks we ought to go. He talked with a person who went there with only a couple weeks to live.

We agreed it depends upon the outcome tomorrow. That includes results of blood work. We will not be in favor of more chemo if red results are not up. If still down, it would dictate the need for more transfusions and the risk gets higher each time. Am extremely concerned with possibility of infection resulting from blood transfusions, no matter what I am told. So, will get up early tomorrow morning in order to be at clinic by 9:40 a.m.

My guess is that the doctor will want to put her in the hospital tomorrow morning for another round of chemo. If we agree, then will tell him to schedule for Tuesday morning so can get an early start. Getting to hospital so late means they start late in day and at the end of three days, won't release her until evening.

Another jolt is that her left eye lid is swollen and it looks to me as though something bit her. She has about a half degree of temperature tonight, but don't think there is any reason for concern.

Had time to work on taxes again today, sort of on and off. At no time have I had up to thirty minutes at one time. But I think I'm finally

264

finished. Now, it is a matter of typing up the whole thing, which may take as much as four to six hours.

Dan just called. He is having trouble with his refrigerator which they bought when they moved into house last July. Think we solved the problem over the telephone but believe that defrost control is intermittent. Suggested he call the store where he bought it while it still is in warranty.

I am very apprehensive about wife tonight.

July 15, 1996

Based on a number of things, including conversation with doctor, decided to go ahead with another round of chemo. Wife really made the decision. She has developed so much confidence in the oncologist. Her response when I questioned her decision was that "we shouldn't do anything that would affect our relations with him".

Doctor wanted to put her in hospital for three days, but as I had guessed, she wanted it done at another medical facility. So, we will start tomorrow morning at the facility, rather than the main hospital. If things don't go well, may have to go to the hospital anyway.

Got home about 12:30 p.m. Helper had already gotten here and had started on apartments. We all decided that I could go to Zanesville with Dan and we left about 1:30pm. Michele stayed with Meryl, who had developed a slight temperature. Rather than getting back fairly early, didn't get back until a little after 6 p.m. Had to go to four places to get an emergency prescription filled.

When I arrived home, learned that grandson Nicholas had snuffed a kernel of corn up his nose. They had taken him to hospital. There is a simple way to get it out but he is not old enough yet to understand. You close your mouth, hold the open nostril closed and then blow through the nostril in which the item is lodged. Dan called me from hospital a few minutes ago and they are still waiting for a doctor to see Nicholas. Meantime, Michele went to Dan's home to stay with Riley until they got back.

Then to top things off, wife's temperature went to 99.9. Put in the antibiotics for a swollen eye. Took temperature again at 9 p.m. and it had dropped to 99. Dan called a few minutes ago, saying they were on the way home. All is well except they had a rough day today, as did Michele, who stayed with Riley. She probably won't get home until midnight.

265

Will have to get an early start as we have to be at annex by 10 a.m. for first intravenous chemo. Then back again Wednesday and again Thursday. Next, the shots begin on Friday. Neupogen for ten days, and Epogen three times a week for a month and probably more.

July 16, 1996

Took Meryl for her first session of this fourth round of chemo. One of prescriptions doctor gave me was for Epogen, the red blood assist and which would have cost about $1,600.

Michele volunteered to bring Meryl home when chemo was finished, while I took off for Wright-Pat to get several prescriptions filled. Today was payday and the base was in turmoil. Took almost two hours to get prescriptions filled.

Helper worked today and most of trimming has been finished for this time. Still haven't mowed grass as it has hardly grown. Except for a couple of spots of rain last weekend which hardly got ground wet, things are still dry.

Another chemo treatment tomorrow morning. Then, the shots begin again. So far, Meryl seems to be holding up okay, but I am worried about blood counts and need for transfusion.

Went to grocery tonight and among other things, bought a pork loin which I had sliced with the intention of broiling. By the time I got back, it was too late. I heated up some barbecue, prepared a cucumber salad and baked a couple of potatoes.

July 17, 1996

Arrived at medical facility at about 9:45 a.m., but they took her early. I questioned nurse about the red blood not coming back up to normal and asked if iron was okay. She did a print-out from yesterday and found iron was very low. Had asked about this Monday and was told it was all right. Didn't really believe this, but figured that I may have been overly concerned. But today, I was given a prescription for ferrous sulfate, which I started giving her this afternoon.

Several times we have asked about the leg pains returning and have no satisfaction or solutions besides medication. Meryl has been frustrated.

Sometimes I wonder if all the tests really mean anything. If they do, it's almost like a computer scan, instead of a person able to analyze and diagnose. The more I learn, the more I question. The whole system seems too robotic.

Now have two additional medications, the eye ointment and iron. Think I am becoming a little bewildered with it all, but have updated the medical schedule again.

Even though wife said she wasn't hungry, she cleaned up a pork chop, salad and white corn. But then, so did I.

Perhaps I get carried away with all this description of the days as they pass. But in a way, I'm paying back the years she sacrificed for her husband and family.

July 18, 1996

It has not been the best of days. Yes, this round of chemo is over and I am regretting I did not follow my gut feeling. It has not gone too well this time around.

No appetite or energy and temperature has been climbing for three days since chemo began. Finally tonight, temperature rose to 100.6. I have been told by doctor that the danger point was 100.5. Called the doctor at home and told him what was happening. He didn't seem alarmed, as he said it was too early, that the temperature would be a problem in ten to fourteen days during the critical period after chemo. He said to give her a couple of Tylenol every four hours and call nurse for blood work in morning.

I mentioned that nurses were not available very early, but I would take her to another medical facility in the morning. They would do blood work there.

Meantime, lunch was a little Jello with fruit that I made yesterday and dinner was tomato soup.

It is now 9:10 p.m. and I will take her temperature again in about ten minutes. Am hoping that it will not be any higher. She made constant trips to bathroom today as there seems to be a build-up of fluid. I got portable potty out of basement, as she will probably have to get up during night several times and might not be able to make it to bathroom. The potty is beside the bed so it will take little time or effort. I will set the alarm for midnight to give her more medication.

Have been unable to devote time to anything this week except taking care of patient. Have always promised myself that I would do this if a problem ever occurred. However, I must confess that I am going though a constant state of anxiety, depression and stress as there is hardly any time away from direct contact with the situation. It's also frustrating not to be able to find time for anything else. I think that worry tempers my ability to concentrate on what I should be doing.

My concern right now is to get the fever down and hope that a trip to the hospital will not be necessary. Got home from clinic today about noon and house was cool. She was cold so I turned on the furnace. When temperature got up to 84, she became comfortable and I was perspiring. Have just taken her temperature again and it has dropped so I have a feeling of relief.

July 19, 1996

Wife's temperature last night had dropped about a degree by midnight. I had set the alarm and got up at a little after midnight to put in eye ointment and two Tylenol's. By this morning, temperature was back to normal. Still no appetite this morning.

Arrived at medical facility by about 10:30 a.m. for blood work. Her temperature was below normal. Lunch was part of a strawberry Ensure. Arrived home about 3 p.m. She still was not hungry, but had to take pills. Some she had to skip because it was too late. She ate a little Jello. By supper time, her temperature was back up to 100.2. No appetite but ate some chicken rice soup.

About an hour later, Michele came in with a pizza. As she started to eat it, wife surprisingly decided she would like a piece. Ate more than two pieces before she quit. I was sure temperature was probably back to normal. Checked it and found it had gone down to 99.1. Will check it again in about fifteen minutes, give her a couple more Tylenol and put in eye ointment. Believe that will suffice for the night.

Dan just called and wanted to know how everything was going. He went to Mansfield today to take depositions. Didn't sound too happy with the outcome. He was putting the boys to bed.

So, this is the story of the ups and downs. Tomorrow morning, a bunch of neighbors have insisted on coming over to do trimming and anything else needed. They said they would not take "No" for an answer.

Another neighbor whom I barely know wants a list by Sunday night of things needed to be done - anything from cleaning toilets, windows and house cleaning. Now just how does someone like me respond?

I have been used to doing for others all my life. Now, people are asking to do for me and it is difficult to handle.

It is time for medication again and another day has ended.

July 20, 1996

Patient feeling a lot better and appetite is back. It's when things get better that I realize how great the stress has been. Still gave a couple more Tylenol this morning and ointment in eye.

I have been moving things to make room for items that will be brought home from Meryl's office. We have to be out by end of month. Will hire a mover, but some things are being done by Dan, Michele and myself. Have moved little items whenever possible. Meantime, medical chores continue.

Have had several people ask about buying her equipment but the offering prices have been ridiculous. However, I may accept just to get rid of it and avoid another task.

One of the neighbors representing the group of people who wanted to come today and help with various tasks, just called. They want to put it off until next week. Not surprised, but good intentions remain.

* * *

DAILY RECORD VIII

July 21, 1996

Michele has taken over the closing out of Meryl's office, but she has great concern with the cosmetics inventory. Although she has been planning and packing for weeks, she wants to wait until the very last day before the final move, because she wants no one to touch the inventory but her.

If the worse comes to worse, I am not adverse to junking the whole thing and writing it off. Felt a little bad as I think spouse could hear what might have sounded like an argument. Will go to church in morning and ask for guidance.

It's past time to cook another ham. Just haven't found exactly what I want. But will bake one in the near future. Worked on taxes today and instead of typing, I found more errors. Tomorrow, if I have time, will go through every form once more and check to see if I've screwed up again.

Dinner tonight was great. Broiled a sirloin, had mashed potatoes and corn. Desert was fruit Jello, with vanilla ice cream. That along with herb iced tea, and there isn't a speck of anything left. Patient seems to be improving. Temperature not totally stable but much closer to normal. Gave second injection of Neupogen today, with eight more to go, one every day. Next Epogen will be Monday.

The prescription for iron has caused a remarkable rise in red blood counts. That was with only one ferrous sulfate pill Wednesday and Thursday. The increase was almost 20% from last Monday to Thursday. The iron I had bought from the vitamin counter was only 40 mg. This prescription is 380. So she is getting almost ten times as much in one pill as I was giving her in ten days.

The doctor did not think initially that iron was deficient. However, the lab report showed it was extremely low. By the way, one hundred of these tablets cost the amazing sum of $1.50. Still needing pain medication at bedtime to smooth out leg pain.

Dan and I moved the baby crib out of our house, and took it to a baby store on consignment. It was set up here at home for the times when the grandsons would stay over. First Riley used it and then Nicholas. Was more difficult than I had anticipated getting it through the doors. We were about an hour just getting the bed out of the house. Then on the way to the store, ran into stopped traffic going to the Parade of Homes, which began today.

Had put out a roast to thaw. When we got back from dropping off baby bed, found that Meryl had come out to kitchen and put roast in electric fry pan. It was cooking. She had also put carrots and potatoes in cold water. Later, I peeled potatoes, skinned carrots and put them into fry pan. She uses it like a roaster. Meat cooked for about three hours, then added veggies which cooked another forty five minutes. Problem is that roast was almost four pounds and there must be over three pounds left.

Meryl's temperature has been better today, although still fluctuating. However, highest today was 99.2 and most of day, was normal. Still gave her a couple of Tylenol at bedtime along with eye ointment. Have not watched Olympiad except for a little tonight. By the time I get to bed, am kind of tired and fall asleep in just a few minutes. Busy day tomorrow but staying busy is good therapy.

July 23, 1996

Had things sort of planned out today, but kept changing agenda as I remembered things I had to do. Instead of moving some items from Meryl's office today, decided to work on taxes. After lunch, finished some errands and picked up some boxes that had been packed.

Remembered that I had an appointment with a reporter for an interview at 2 p.m. Instead of interview lasting only a short time, it went over two hours. He wants to come back once more for additional information. It appears that if and how it is written, will possibly be a magazine article. Have now typed about twelve pages and about half done on taxes. As I recall, still several more pages to go. Expect to finish by Thursday. That will be a big relief.

In just a couple of days, Japanese beetles have stripped about two-thirds of the leaves off the apricot tree. There were hundreds on the tree feasting away. Not only did I use fruit spray but got out wasp and hornet spray and targeted varmints directly.

Michele stopped by and gave her some roast beef to take home. Later, remembered that I forgot to order flowers for an old friend who passed away Sunday. He has had heart problems for a long time. Doctors decided to stop all medication and start over. Was released that afternoon and died that night at home.

Then an old army buddy called me about 8:10 p.m. He was in Columbus with his wife, who is having a pace maker implanted. Expects to go home Thursday. Was telling me he saw a feature program on television recently with some interviews I had done several months ago. Guess I forgot, so I did not get to see it. Said he has always been proud to have been a friend, and that he told everyone who would listen about his regard. We were lieutenants together many years ago.

Wish I could get back to a normal schedule, as I'm perhaps more frustrated than I realized. Critical period yet to come. Hoping this time a transfusion will not be needed. I think the last one could have been avoided if the Epogen and iron had been started sooner, based on information from the drug manufacturer.

July 24, 1996

Gave fifth Neupogen shot today, so if all goes well, five more to go. I suppose that Epogen will continue for the foreseeable future until either chemo stops or blood gets back to normal. Both white and red counts dropped today as critical post-chemo period is near. Still hoping no transfusions needed this time.

Patient has kept me busy today. Last call was forty minutes ago, and have forgotten my train of thought. Been a hectic day. Woke up about 3:30 this morning and couldn't go back to sleep. Went downstairs and took a Melatonin, came back to bed and didn't wake up until almost 8 a.m.. Even then, didn't want to get up.

Later in day, a nurse came. Then someone arrived that Michele had asked to take a look at a walk-in closet in wife's bedroom downstairs to reorganize it.

I took an hour and a half to go to a funeral home and pay respects to an old friend who had a massive heart attack. Stopped at Meryl's office and loaded up a bunch of boxes

Michele and friends had packed last weekend. Went to post office, then picked up results of blood taken this morning and finally home. Left boxes in wagon until tomorrow morning.

After dinner, went out to look at apricot tree and there wasn't a single Japanese Beetle anywhere to be found. They have either left or have met their maker. Supper included the fluffiest mashed potatoes I've ever made. Now have to remember how I did it. Typed more of my tax forms and now have six more pages to go.

My army buddy called again this morning to tell me that he felt vindicated by a newspaper article written about the responsibility shared by those who were around during World War II.

July 25, 1996

Meryl stayed up until 9:25 p.m. which is unusually late for her. But she seems, and my fingers are crossed, to be getting along much better this time. But then, today is day nine since last round of chemo began. Critical period is between ten and fourteen days after so we'll see.

Next blood work will be Friday. If drop is not too drastic, may get by without transfusion. It looks as though the final move for wife's office will be on August 3, as I just today was able to find a mover who could do it on that date. His price was a great deal higher than the usual, but it will be worth it to get it over.

Susan stopped by and brought some food which made up part of supper. In fact, supper was what she brought, plus cold roast beef. Dessert was watermelon. Watched about twenty minutes of the Olympiad tonight. Completed all the tax forms today plus other items that have to accompany the return. This was the most complicated return I have ever had to do. I still have to do the state and local taxes.

Wife seems to be feeling okay today, no temperature and in good spirits. Good appetite and very alert. We are hoping and praying most fervently.

July 26, 1996

Got to the funeral home yesterday afternoon. Sad affair. As I had mentioned, an old friend had a massive heart attack which was brought on by the problem of a dog going out of the house and not coming back. His wife had heard a howl and ran outside to see what was wrong. He ran out also. They found the dog dead, but didn't find out what happened. Within a few minutes after they took the dog inside, my friend had a massive heart attack. Never knew what hit him. So his wife had to bury him and the dog. Strange how things happen.

Today, worked on state tax which is now done and will finish local tax tomorrow. Also, worked on an engineering report for Dan on the inspection I did for him on the dryer at a laundromat..

Went to wife's office today and left a bunch of boxes which Michele and some friends are going to pack tomorrow through the weekend. Brought back all they had packed earlier this week, and all is put away. Can't believe that I had enough space.

Movers will take care of big stuff on August 3, which is the last day to move without paying another month's rent. Space has been leased to others already. Dan is renting a truck Saturday to remove the remaining smaller items.

Also, mowed after dinner tonight and finished the apartments. Got a little done at the house and will try to finish that tomorrow. As I look back on all that I've done today, it's hard to believe that one person can do that much in one day. And I had plenty of medical work to do as is the case every day. Just put wife to bed after providing medication, took temperature which was normal and put in eye ointment. Eye seems to be back almost to normal except that there is a sty or something which may have to be removed.

Today is day number ten since last round of chemo began, so it is the first day of the critical period. It continues for the next three to six days. Appetite still good but have fingers crossed.

July 27, 1996

Not complicated, but a non stop day. Got up this morning about 6:45 with usual medication, breakfast, etc. Meantime, was getting laundry together on which I had gotten behind. Did four loads of laundry and they were big loads. Nurse came and tried to get blood without success, as Metaport didn't work. Finally, after needle was placed in second port, blood began to flow.

While she was doing that, a roofing man arrived to give me an estimate on replacing garage roof as well as new flashing around dormers of house. Have developed a bad leak on two of them and the plaster in house has been damaged.

Next, got lunch, made huge dish of cherry Jello with pineapple, apricots, fruit cocktail and walnuts. It was so heavy that I had difficulty trying to hold it up with one hand. At same time, was looking at state tax return.

After lunch, put some laundry away and hung up other items to dry. Went to grocery, then post office and stopped at lab to pick up blood report. For the eleventh day after chemo start, Meryl is much better than last time. Last month on the eleventh day, she was in hospital getting a blood transfusion.

Changed clothes and got out tractor but first, took liver out of freezer for supper. While I was mowing, Dan came up the drive in the biggest truck you can imagine. Told me it was the only one he could find. We cleared out his drum set, skis, guns, tennis rackets and other items which he took home. Needed the space to make room for items coming out of the office. He is going to start moving things tomorrow morning rather early. I have to get breakfast and give medication, so will have to join him later. However, he has three or four people helping so it shouldn't be too bad. Part of the things comes here, part to Michele and part to his house. Dan's pole barn is coming in handy.

For supper tonight, had broiled liver, mashed potatoes, pita bread and Jello. Have gotten to where my mashed potatoes are a gourmet's (Me) delight. But I shouldn't take credit as my wife showed me how to do it.

Called Wright-Pat and left prescription for eight different drugs. Will be ready tomorrow, but am not planning to go until Sunday. Day is finally winding down. Once more, I can't believe how much I've gotten done. Did not stop the whole day or tonight. Am a little tired. Wife still getting a little pain medication at bedtime.

July 28, 1996

Things still look good, but am very apprehensive about red blood counts. Am terribly worried about more transfusions as I just don't have any real faith about the validity of testing of blood. Too many uncertainties and am afraid of new health problems coming from blood.

Another unbelievable day today. At exactly 8 a.m., neighbors and friends began showing up to work on yard. Within a half hour, there were fourteen people pulling weeds out of the flower circle. I was in and out of the house, but I hauled all the weeds in the wheel barrow and threw them over the bank next to the creek. Lost track of just how many trips I made. By 11 a.m., all was finished. And just in time as Dan came up the hillside drive in the truck.

He had arrived at wife's office at 7 a.m. Had one of my brothers, two nephews and sister-in-law help load and unload. Took about an hour to unload, then he went on to Michele's where he unloaded the stuff she will store, took the rest to his house. Meantime, noticed that there was a hole in the ground in front of the house and sure enough, it was a yellow jacket nest. Waited until almost dark when the wasps were all in the nest and then went out to pour a chemical compound into the hole.

Lunch was late due to all the activity, didn't finish until about 2:30. Am not sure where we are going to put all the various things. Right now, house is sort of packed. Next Saturday, movers will get rest of stuff and that chore will be over. Today was Neupogen shot number nine. Tomorrow will be the tenth, and hope the last, for this chemo series. Epogen however goes on for awhile until red count comes up.

Nurse sort of gave away something. When I asked about the need for iron, I was told all was fine. However, without telling me, an iron test was ordered with the blood that had been taken. That's when I was given the prescription for iron.

The nurse asked me how Meryl was taking the iron after having seen the report. I asked her for a copy and she gave it to me. Iron was down over seventy five percent, so anemia was bound to be a problem. Sometimes, one needs to ask obvious questions. Have reached a point now where I understand the lab reports much better. Am still giving her supplements. As counts come up, then am easing off on supplements.

Went out this afternoon to post office, grocery and another stop. Was gone about an hour and a half but all was well when I got back. Am beginning to feel that Dan and Michele want to help take care of their mother. But neither one has the time nor should they take the time from their own busy schedules. So, must still feel that responsibility is pretty much all mine.

Come Monday, will begin search again for someone who would be available to stay overnight on occasion. I'd rather not have to depend on kids or relatives. They mean well, but the spirit and the time are not in agreement.

Mashed potatoes again tonight. They have become addictive.

July 29, 1996

Time flies when you don't want it to and it drags when you want it to fly. That's not really good because we should never wish time away, no matter how boring or unexciting. Went to Wright-Pat today. Left early and got back in afternoon. Had a real slowdown west of Springfield, with traffic stopped because only one lane was open and crazy drivers were all trying to get in the same lane. So lost perhaps ten minutes and still got home in time. Found both Michele and sister-in-law here.

Took patient's temperature, pulse, blood pressure and gave eye ointment - just to name a few of the things that needed doing. Had all medication laid out before I left and marked, so all they needed to do was take them to her at the prescribed time. Dan had been there with Riley for a short time this morning, but I know that he had a golf date this afternoon.

Dinner tonight was spaghetti with a sauce. Made a salad which wife could not eat, as during what they call the critical period, no fresh fruit or vegetables. Afraid of bacterial infection from the mist that is sprayed at stores. Michele had time to come back and had supper with us.

July 30, 1996

Nurse was here to take blood. I picked up lab report in the afternoon. Red count dropped again, which I hoped would not happen. Told doctor that count was so low when last round of chemo started that it was almost a sure bet for a transfusion. Was hoping that iron and Epogen would change that.

Received telephone call from nurse saying doctor had ordered a transfusion for tomorrow morning so will take her to hospital. This is what I have been dreading. Really would like to have waited another day but the way the nurse put it, if anything happened, it would be entirely my responsibility. So, I don't feel that I'm qualified to take on that kind of stress in spite of my apprehension.

Workers are coming tomorrow to redo closet, something Michele ordered. Called them and asked if they could come two hours earlier. I felt I could come home to meet them and get back to hospital before transfusion was finished. I cleared out the closet and took down the shelves.

Michele called from Toledo and I had to tell her the bad news. Am prepared to tell the doctor that we want no more chemo now until blood gets back to normal range. However, wife's desires come first. Anemia causes a feeling of being tired and feeling cold, even when it's hot. But I was still hoping for improvement. So now, all is quiet except the keyboard.

July 31, 1996

Seems that the pace is getting breath taking. Or is it just my breath. The day starts as it did yesterday about 5 a.m. for me and then it goes non stop until time to sleep. Didn't really need to get up that early but woke up, couldn't go back to sleep so got up.

Took care of medication, temperature and breakfast a little earlier than usual so we could get off to the hospital just before 9 a.m. However, it was a long day with a nurse who just wasn't with it. When the transfusion was finished, she took out needles in Metaport but forgot to put in special medication. So, she had to put new needles back in and do what she had forgotten. If I hadn't asked, she probably wouldn't have done it. But the syringes were lying on the table and when I asked her about it, then she admitted forgetting.

Had arrived at hospital early. Had to wait almost an hour before anything started, even though no doctors were involved and arrangements had been made yesterday. I couldn't get away until about 11 a.m.

Man to redo closet arrived at 12:30 instead of noon as arranged. I had cleared everything including old shelves so all he had to do was put on brackets and hang shelves. He was finished in about forty minutes, instead of two hours.

The roofer arrived at 12:30 exactly, the time set for the appointment. He gave me an estimate which I found acceptable and signed the contract. The new roof on the garage will cost almost as much as building the entire garage cost originally. The garage was added in about 1972 or so. The roof has lasted twenty-four years which isn't bad. The original roof on the house which is slate and shingles has been on since 1927. They don't make them like that anymore.

Arrived back at hospital thinking patient would be finished shortly after I got there. No such luck. They had started real late on first blood packet and had just started the second when I arrived. Didn't get home until after 5 p.m.

Started supper which was simple tonight as one of our neighbor food providers brought over homemade vegetable soup and cantaloupe last night. I ate the cantaloupe as she can't have either fruit or vegetables fresh. We had vegetable soup and hot dog for supper. She finally went to bed about 9:30 after sleeping most of the day at hospital. Had a little time to type about a page on report for Dan.

Am still upset about incompetence of nurse who provided support for Meryl today. Am very apprehensive about infection as a result of not paying attention to what she was doing and worse, not practicing good sanitary procedures. So am keeping my fingers crossed about the outcome of all this. Wish now that I had refused this round of chemotherapy. She was feeling so much better. May just be edgy but have a gut feeling that something is wrong.

Nurse is coming tomorrow morning to take blood as doctor now has to decide if she is to get a platelet transfusion also. If so, then another trip to the hospital. The red counts went up just a little today before the transfusion, but platelet count really dropped. Am hoping that it will be up tomorrow morning. Meantime, she has gone to bed and all is quiet so time for me to go to bed. Since weeding of the circle by neighbors last Saturday, have had several comments on how nice it looks. I think it's just the contrast between nothing visible but weeds, and now the weeds are gone and the various plantings are visible. Too often, the obvious is not appreciated until it is lost and then becomes visible again.

August 1, 1996

Red counts and platelets dropped a little more since yesterday. Doctor's nurse called in late in PM and he wants another blood sample taken tomorrow morning. If platelets are down more, then have to take her tomorrow for a platelets transfusion. Am keeping fingers crossed and hoping no platelets will be needed. Also, my concern continues about last transfusion, as well as Metaport, as a source of infection.

In the morning, yard helper came and I had him trim with mower and pick up a number of limbs which had blown off in the storm yesterday. Some of the limbs off the walnut trees were pretty good size and heavy.

After lunch, I went to post office, then to wife's office. I loaded a bunch of clothes from the walk-in closet in the bedroom, which she maintained on the nights she stayed there. Couple more good loads and the movers coming Sunday will finish up. The house here, however, is a mess with things stuck all over the place. The buzzer just rang and went down-stairs for final medication of the day.

August 3, 1996

Wife is not feeling well at all. I see a steady deterioration in her condition. Am now more convinced than ever that should have waited for last round of chemo. Also, now wondering if I should have waited another day on transfusion.

All this uncertainty and the weight of responsibility is becoming terribly stressful. Feel as though if we had waited for another round of chemo, when she was feeling better, we could have gone to San Diego for treatment. She might have had some days she could have enjoyed.

Now, temperature is very erratic, from above to below normal. She is losing weight and appetite is gone. However, she has been fairly interested in final move of furniture and equipment from her office today. This was the deadline for moving out. Am not sure that the closing of office is not a morale factor. It's just one more psychological factor in the finality of this disease.

Pain is now a constant condition every night and am using pain salve plus medication. Am in a constant state of apprehension and grief. And nothing that I can do about it. It's just that I feel so bad for her and she has such a great fear of dying. Can't blame her, as we had looked forward so much to being able to take time to do some things we had always wanted to do.

What bothers me, too, is the terrible responsibility that is placed on me with so little knowledge of the disease and treatment. At this point, believe that treatment is worse than the disease and that what is available in the way of conventional treatment causes terrible pain, suffering and nausea. Worse, it is not a cure.

Perhaps it's best to treat the points causing the problems, such as the lesion on the spine that's causing pain in her back and legs. Then, let the disease take its course. Am also realizing the uncertainty that many families must go through. The dilemma is terrible. I know what I would do for myself in these circumstances, but how do I know what is best?

If we opt for one alternative and it doesn't work, then we must ask whether we did the right thing or if it would have been different if something else were done.

August 5, 1996

Yesterday was not too good. Wife continues to experience varying temperatures, from below normal to as much as almost two degrees of fever. She still is smoking. Residue has gotten so bad in her bathroom that I told her yesterday I was going to buy a deionizer for bath room because everyone was complaining when they got near the door. That set off a response that amounts to punishment by silence. She isn't feeling well. But I think now she knows she can't hide her smoking, and she is embarrassed.

Next appointment is next Monday at which time the doctor will want to start the next round of chemo. With the way things have gone this time, I am absolutely opposed. Don't think she will survive another without intensive hospitalization.

Taxes are in the mail, office move is over and now, have to figure out how to unclutter a house that is bursting at the seams with stuff for which there is no room. My concern is growing. She has deteriorated since the transfusion and can't help feel that she has developed something new. Temperature indicates an infection or something. That is upsetting.

August 7, 1996

Wife woke me up early this morning. She could not breath. I boiled some water in a pan, added Vicks and had her breath it. After about five 5 minutes, she was better. I called the fire department to ask where I could buy some oxygen. The firefighters offered to bring over a bottle until I could make other arrangements, and they arrived very quickly.

After we put Meryl on oxygen, she began feeling much better. I called doctor and made an appointment for 1:30 p.m. They took a chest x-ray, and found the tumor was difficult to define. Where it had been a sharp, well-defined area originally, there was now a scattered mass.

I think, however, she has come down with some kind of flu or sinus infection. But the doctor is concerned that the tumor is blocking her air passage.

At the hospital tomorrow, they are going to pass a tube into her lung to see what is going on. It's called a bronchoscopy. Started her on antibiotics today, but instructions seem to conflict with some of the drugs she is using. Need to find a good pharmacist who knows drugs.

It is after 9 p.m. and all is quiet except my pecking away at the keyboard. Right now, don't have to describe my cooking prowess as have not been cooking very much. It's been canned chicken rice soup for the most of the past two days, same today and fruit Jello. Plus a whole lot of pills. Can't believe the amount of medication she is taking. Over $15,000 worth of medication given to her at the hospital.

Talked with doctor today and asked if there could be some time off from chemo. He said he has waited a month for some people, and there is no reason why it couldn't happen again. So, if she feels better, she will be able to keep a dental appointment and still have time to go to Mexico for the three weeks treatment there. All now depends on what they find.

Michele left for Toledo this afternoon and will be there until Friday. That is where her company headquarters is located. She has to make a presentation. Dan stopped by tonight and stayed until about 8:30 p.m. Think he is quite worried about the uncertainty. Glad that I insisted on the pneumonia shots last January. It supposedly carries an immunity for about eight years.

News seems to be always stressful these days. Or perhaps it is just my own perceptions and apprehensions coming out.

* * *

DAILY RECORD IX

August 9, 1996

Meryl's breathing was very difficult when she awakened this morning. I went to the fire department and had two oxygen bottles filled, so she could go back on oxygen.

Nurse came to take blood, but decided instead that we should go to the hospital immediately. I called the fire department and talked to the chief, who sent an ambulance to take Meryl to the hospital on a non-emergency basis.

I followed in my car and arrived shortly after they moved her into a room. Doctor had made arrangements for admission. I answered the usual battery of questions about medication and history. I was prepared, because I had taken with me a computer copy of the medication schedules that I used to keep track of the times and amounts of doses. I gave it to the doctor in attendance, a very nice, concerned young intern.

It looks like they are going to take more X-rays, cat scans, MRI and am not sure what else. Since today is Friday, probably won't start radiation treatment until Monday. The radiation section is usually closed on Saturday and Sunday. They won't mark her or start radiation until other tests are done. Meantime, she is on oxygen with an oxygen blood saturation device attached to her. Also, IV was started and guess they will keep her on it. Metaport will take fluids coming in but won't work to get blood.

I just have this totally helpless feeling that everything is out of control.

Finally left hospital about 9 p.m. Michele was still there. Dan thought he would come down later, even though it was already late. Tried to talk him out of it but he insists. Am very tired tonight, as usual, but probably won't sleep well.

August 10, 1996

Very restless night. Got up, had a quick bite and then went to hospital. Wife was asleep when I got there, so just sat down and didn't wake her. I was told she had been awake most of the night with some of the tests that were not completed until after midnight.

She is in terrible pain in right hip and can't be moved except to be lifted. At times, she is unable to get out of bed and has to use a bedpan. Just the slightest movement and she screams with the pain.

More tests are to be completed today. She is no longer able to use a wheelchair. I also now am concerned that lying on her back all the time is going to cause fluid to accumulate in her lungs.

Stayed all day at the hospital, but did leave for a short time in the afternoon to run an errand. When I got back, we were told that they found a hairline fracture in the right hip which was caused by a lesion. It was in a non-weight bearing area.

They were going to start radiation on the hip and had already started radiation on the lung. At this point, my confidence is gone, but I can't let her know that. I have this feeling that everything is now being attended from a panic point of view. Try this and try that, but really feel that things have gone too far. But, I want and must feel that something positive is going to happen.

Left hospital about 10 p.m. I'm not looking forward to a restful night. Michele still was at the hospital when I left. Needless to say, everything is now secondary to my wife's situation. Can't believe how quickly things have changed.

August 11, 1996

Day is beautiful, even if it can't be enjoyed. Michele was at the hospital when I arrived and was going to stay for perhaps another hour.

Situation is not good. About a degree of temperature, constant pain and continued difficulty breathing. It appears that cancer is coming back and more tumors are forming. But doctors don't seem to know for sure. They think that good cells are being attacked, causing inflammation. Meryl is getting an anti-inflammatory drug to combat that development.

Several visitors during morning and afternoon, including a sister-in law, plus a niece and her husband. Michele returned about 4:30 p.m. Only times I have been outside today were when I arrived at the hospital and left. It's one of those days when I am very discouraged and feel very hopeless about everything.

Took the Sunday paper to the hospital where I read it. It seems that I barely had time to finish the paper between the company visits. In the room next door, there was a black patient and, late in the afternoon, they had a sort of revival in the room. Nurse told me that in another room on the other side of the hospital, over thirty families were having a religious ceremony for another patient. While the one next door was fairly vocal, understand that the big one was really loud. Hospital didn't seem to know what to do about it. Seems the establishment and God are not compatible these days.

My wife was unable to rest until all the noise ended. Got home late and my feeling of hopelessness continues.

August 12, 1996

Time moves rapidly but it seems those we love endure only a moment in the flight of time. It is true so many times that we look back and wish we had done this or that when the opportunity was there.

Wife was feeling a little better today, with breathing a little easier. Read for a little while, as she was asleep when I got there. Then I fell asleep on and off for about forty-five minutes.

Dan arrived about 1 p.m. as they were taking her down to X-ray. We went out for a bite to eat. Things seemed to be okay so we left about 4 p.m. Found out that Michele could not go to the hospital tonight. I checked and found out that Meryl was to get a transfusion this evening. Seems that red count, hemoglobin and hematocrit have all dropped. Platelets are fine however. They don't know why this has happened. I was about to go back, but she insisted I stay home and rest.

Susan came to the house in the evening with both boys, and brought a plate of meat, mashed potatoes, corn on cob and salad.

I am very distressed with what is happening to Meryl. Can't shake this feeling that cancer has suddenly started to spread and it is now out of control. She still is on oxygen and having trouble breathing. Throughout my lifetime, I have gone through many periods of stress including wars, but can't remember anything like this.

I am extremely worried, but my real sorrow is for her and all the suffering and fear she is experiencing. Somewhere, there must be something better..

August 13, 1996

Meryl was dozing when I arrived at the hospital. Nurse awakened her. Just before lunch, they announced they were taking her for an X-ray of her hip and then would give radiation treatment. I asked when she would have lunch. They decided they should get her a tray of food immediately. They did.

At times, everybody is so busy that patient care is not all that great. I have tremendous concern when I am not there to make sure that each problem is addressed. She ate lunch, and it was a good thing. They took her out about 12:30 and she didn't get back until almost 4 p.m.

I finally went down to the radiation department to find her. By the time I got there, nobody knew where she was. One nurse told me that she was lying on a cot in a corner for quite awhile. That also happened yesterday. I don't intend to let that happen again, because I will go with her each time she is taken out of the room from now on. If this happens again, I will do whatever is necessary to prevent it. Besides, the cot is hard and it's cold in the area where they shove her to wait.

She enjoyed supper, which among other items included mashed potatoes, gravy, liver and onions. Believe that her appetite is coming back. Michele came in about 6 p.m. and I left shortly after. Went home, had a bite to eat.

I called Dan to see if he had been able to print out his tax return, and told him I would be out in a few minutes to review it for him.

Tomorrow, will get up, go to hospital again and wait to see what develops.

August 14, 1996

I have been awakening early every morning. Today it was about 5 a.m. Some mornings it's as early at 3:30 a.m.

Not a good day except that the red blood counts made a dramatic jump upward. They were worried about internal bleeding, but that proved to be a false possibility. Stool test was negative. It was dark and has been, with red counts down. My guess was that stool's dark color was because of the iron she has been taking.

Those are the two items of good news. However, the hip pain becomes unbearable when she moves. They took her for an MRI last night at 11 p.m. She didn't want to go, and got very little sleep all night.

Her appearance was not good this morning. Not to belabor the point too long, they finally closed the door and put a sign on it that patient needed quiet time. Doctors were in several times.

The last doctor was an orthopedic specialist with the bad news. The right hip has a slight fracture on which there can be no surgery. He feels that it will heal in a few weeks but pain will continue. A lesion caused by cancer in the bone resulted in the fracture, he said. They are going to start radiation treatment on the hip, also, but no time table just now. Major problem is that one thing after another is going wrong.

She is losing not only hope but has an increasing degree of despair. She is also very "scared", which is the word she used in telling doctor how she felt. Guess we can do nothing but hope and pray. I do both constantly.

Got home and found that tree men had been here. Problem is that the yard has a couple of eighteen-inch limbs which were dropped and left there. Roofers are supposed to start in next few days and haven't heard from them. Still another opportunity. Think I could do with a few less opportunities.

Still awakening early every morning. Getting behind on some things, and worry about that, but nothing urgent right now. There is a possibility I will go to Wright-Pat either Friday or Saturday.

August 15, 1996

Blood work today has all the red blood count, hematocrit and hemoglobin in the bottom of the normal range. This is the first time since February this has been so. Of course, she had another transfusion night before last so that probably helped. The hip is not painful except when she moves a certain way. Then when attendants are careless, she will scream with pain. The agony only lasts a few seconds, but it has gotten so bad that she does not want to move at all. To transfer her from the bed and move her to X-ray takes four people. She has a pad below her and is lifted with the pad, so she is able to stay immobile.

They have doubled her pain medicine which keeps her in a sort of drugged state.

Today they marked her right hip and started radiation treatments there. This is in addition to the lung, which they started radiating when she entered the hospital. They say the fracture will heal by itself, but will require at least a couple of weeks before it starts feeling better.

Don't know what time it is now, but must be near midnight. Will plan to go to Wright-Pat Saturday morning to pick up prescriptions.

August 16, 1996

Dan was at the hospital when I arrived this morning, but left shortly afterwards. Meryl seemed to be a little better today. Nurse gave me copy of today's blood work. For the first time since February, red counts are all in the bottom of the normal range. In fact, most of the results are now in the normal range. They stopped the Epogen today as they don't want the counts to get above normal.

A new problem has developed in that both arms were swollen yesterday. The left arm went back to normal while the other remained obviously swollen. Called it to doctor's attention and they immediately took her off all IV's. This morning her arms looked almost normal, but they are trying to figure out if there is a clot causing problem.

Frankly, I think it is the Metaport, which has been nothing but a problem since it was surgically installed. Is it possible that clots are forming in Metaport itself or in the tubing that goes into the vein from the Metaport? They did some kind of sonic scan, but could find nothing. So far today, they have given her radiation treatments on lung and on hip, then next she went to sonic test. Finally, at 6 p.m., they took her down for a chest X-ray. I went along each time to make sure that she wasn't left lying around as happened twice this week.

Although she seems to be feeling better, except for the extreme pain in the right hip because of the fracture, she doesn't have much appetite. I think part of problem is that because she has to be lifted in and out of bed, there may be a psychological block to eating. Plus, having her always lying on her back bothers me. She has several nurses however who are absolute jewels and take exceptional care of her. I am quite thankful about that.

Finally left hospital about 7 p.m. Don't feel that I've accomplished much. It's been a long day and think I will stop now. Will hit the sack early in order to get an early start tomorrow for Wright-Patterson AFB..

August 17, 1996

Stopped at hospital after I returned from Wright-Pat and found they had tried to call me on an emergency. They felt it was urgent to place a filter in main vein going to lungs. Dan gave the authorization. Meryl was perfectly capable of making the decision, except for being doped up with pain killers. She seems to be a little better, but far from anything close to normal. Her strength is gone and the constant lying on her back is not good. No radiation today as that part of hospital closes on weekends unless there is an emergency.

August 18, 1996

Went to Mass this morning and then to hospital. Not a good day as kidney problems are now beginning to develop. The alternatives are either a tremendous amount of liquid by mouth or else back on an IV. I am very apprehensive of going back on IV, as this caused swelling problem before. Besides, high tech Metaport has not worked for several days, nothing is being done about that. The nurse said the surgeon would probably look at it Monday. He is not available on weekends except in emergencies.

Meryl is getting weaker each day and my apprehension grows greater each day. Susan went to a function of some sort so Dan spent the day at home and was unable to go to hospital. Michele called and said she was not feeling well, so advised her not to come to hospital.

I am at home now, wearing a hospital outfit a friend gave me several years ago, while I am doing a laundry of clothing and bed linen. I will call the hospital about midnight to find out what latest lab work results are.

I must have faith and believe a better life is ahead for all of us.

August 19, 1996

I was told they were going to take out the Metaport this morning. I was disappointed later when they put it off until afternoon. Radiation treatments today. We left the room at 11:10 a.m., and returned about 11:30 a.m. No more delays or being left in a corner. Lunch was late, but she was able to eat much more than usual. Guess they had a delicious pot roast.

The surgeon came in about 1:30 p.m. and let me watch the Metaport removal. He was worried about my having a weak stomach. I told him that I had seen far worse on the battlefield. Watched the whole thing almost in an abstract manner, including the pulling out of the port and tubing, then watched the suturing. Took eleven stitches to close the wound. They wanted to observe her to make sure all was okay. Intern came in and went over three pages of instruction details. This young man has been outstanding and has devoted a lot of time which he does not do for all patients. I think he has taken a genuine interest in my wife.

Ambulance was scheduled to leave at 6 p.m. to take her home. She can not go by car because of the hip, yet I am to bring her to the hospital tomorrow morning by car for more radiation treatments. Ambulance didn't arrive until 6:45 p.m. I went out to the desk and had them call before that. It appeared they had forgotten. Two calls later finally found them at the entrance. The two young men were really personable and caring.

Got her in bed at home finally about 8 p.m. I went out for prescriptions and some groceries. Am pooped. Will go to bed very quickly tonight.

August 20, 1996

Today was another day that went literally non-stop. Got patient up about 8 a.m. for medication and breakfast. Took longer to get out to car than I figured because of pain in fractured hip. But things went pretty well and we arrived for 11 a.m. appointment five minutes early. Forgot to take a pillow for wheel chair so it wasn't the most comfortable ride. However, they took her as soon as we arrived.

Radiologist saw her immediately after radiation treatment, and we were back home before noon. Either we are getting preferential treatment or we are just lucky.

Order for dinner tonight was liver, onions, mashed potatoes and gravy. Got back a plate with just a little gravy residue. Think she is getting her appetite back again. Had to revise the medication sheet again. This was revision number eight. Changed the format of the layout to make it more understandable.

August 21, 1996

It's been a very stressful day. Wife was in terrible pain, even with heavy medication. She did not know what day it was or the time of day. It was very difficult getting her out of bed and to the car for trip to hospital. However, finally managed, got there and took wheelchair out of trunk, got her in it and finally to radiation about ten minutes before appointment. They took her right away but it was a half hour before they brought her back.

Staff was not happy because they complained that it took twenty minutes to get her out of the wheelchair and onto the table. So, we ended up with approval for an ambulance to transport her to and from the hospital.

Last night, I believe Meryl went to the bathroom by herself, and I'm sure that she fell. Bathroom sink was full of cigarette ashes. She also wanted to go to the bathroom when we returned from the hospital today. I believe it was for the purpose of a cigarette. In the process, she fell again and scraped both knees. I also think she injured both her left ankle as well as her left wrist. With so much medication, I doubt if any pain in those areas is noticed.

For lunch, Meryl wanted cream cheese, olives and some Jello. Didn't have any Jello so gave her some cold pineapple. Also made a sandwich on wheat bread out of the cheese mix with a slice of tomato.

No shot today, but one tomorrow. Then not again until Monday. Last antibiotics will be Sunday afternoon. Red counts have been going back down since they stopped the Epogen shots, but I was told to start them again Wednesday. Back to schedule again of Monday, Wednesday and Friday until red counts get back up. They are not bad, in fact higher than they have been in weeks. But with the radiation, both white and red counts will drop.

Went out tonight, while Michele was here, and bought bed pads and a bed pan. Couldn't find bed pads but did find chair pads. Same thing only smaller. Needed two pads to cover area.

Sister-in-law also baked a delicious apple pie, but everyone was too full to sample except me. Some things I never turn down, one being apple pie.

Tomorrow should be kind of a snap, since I won't have to do anything to get to hospital or back again. Ambulance will handle that. The nurse comes at 9 a.m. to take blood. They are concerned now about possible renal problems. The kidneys and liver can only take so much, before all the radiation and chemo have their affect. This treatment may be the accepted procedure in conventional medicine but it destroys any quality of life for whatever time remains. If this ever happens to me, I will let the disease put me under before it comes to this.

Why live and suffer in this way? But there is comfort in knowing she is still here. And there is agony watching her live a life, or rather endure a life of pain.

August 22, 1996

Nurse came this morning, blood pressure, then blood for lab work. Ambulance arrived with a guy and a girl medics. It was sort of uneven, as she had a little trouble carrying her end of the weight. To get Meryl out of bed, we had to put a sheet under her and lift her with the sheet. The girl decided to get on the bed and lift from that end. However, she didn't bother to remove her shoes and left marks on white sheet. Hard to believe a medic would do something like that. In getting her out, they left long black marks on the white hall walls where they rubbed the stretcher, and they scraped paint off the door.

That seemed strange, since Meryl can't weigh more than 100 pounds. I wondered what they do with someone really heavy. Finally got her loaded and I rode with them. Got there just on time and they took her immediately, finishing in about fifteen minutes.

Back at home, I decided to get involved to prevent more damage. Also, I took off my shoes and took the bed side while I let the female medic move wife's legs. However, instead of moving her legs as we moved her, the female medic didn't move at all so hip was jarred with a lot of pain in the process. Guess my wish at this point is that they don't send her again.

There are nine more radiation treatments left but I am hoping the hip will begin to heal and be less painful so we don't need the ambulance each day.

Fixed a half barbecue sandwich on wheat for lunch, as well as black cherry fruit Jello. She was not too hungry but finished what was on her plate. Michele came over for supper of beef and noodles, mashed potatoes, salad and apple pie. The three of us polished off everything.

Michele stayed here while I went to Dan's and helped him install a defrost assembly in their new refrigerator. Only took about twenty minutes. Then went to Michele's where I dropped off her birthday present, which was an outdoor gas barbecue grill. It has been in the back of my station wagon for several weeks. Spent about an hour attempting to assemble it, but had wrong tools. So, will go over this weekend to finish.

Wife had best appetite tonight she has had in several days. Hope things are coming around.

August 23, 1996

Lab report this afternoon showed that all red and white blood counts are now back to normal. I did not give an Epogen shot tonight as instructions from drug manufacturer say to stop when hematocrit reaches 36%. Last Tuesday, it had dropped to about 31%, so began shots on Wednesday. Just one injection got her well into the normal range. Her immune system is down somewhat, however, and liver and kidneys are not performing up to par.

Think a major problem is that she is not drinking enough water to flush them out properly. So, casually mentioned that to both Meryl and Michele tonight. While I was gone on errands, I'm certain Michele discussed this with her. Apparently a great deal of liquid was consumed while I was gone for about two hours.

Another consideration is that she is taking Bactrim, which is an antibiotic which should be taken with lots of water. If not, crystals can form in the kidneys, similar to problems formerly related to Sulfa. I'm hoping the liquid problem is solved.

I had time today to spend an hour on medical bills, and it is a nightmare. Must have at least two hundred forms from hospitals, clinics, Medicare, and Aetna. My attempt to correlate them was not totally a successful effort. Many items are missing so will have to make several phone calls to get the information needed to pay the amounts due.

There is lots of talk about what is wrong with so many things. My observation is that everything has been made so complicated, it increases the amount of time and work to the point it is almost impossible to get anything done. Have we become so bogged down in paperwork that we no longer have time to really understand the problems we have created? I once stated in a speech. "Too often, today's problems are a result of yesterday's solutions". Is our memory so short that we can't comprehend this?

August 24, 1966

Today is Saturday and it has been another long day. Put together a packet for the clinic near San Diego and will mail it Monday. Wife has been really out of it today. Problems include breathing, which I think comes from lying on her back most of the time, uncontrolled bowels and total lethargy. I sensed she was in something like a semi-coma, but Dan believes her condition resulted from the accumulation of all the narcotic-type drugs she has been taking.

One nurse in the hospital gave her real heavy doses of a morphine-base drug whenever she wanted it. I did not voice an opinion, or I would have had both spouse and the nurse on my back.

I have read that anyone who lacks mobility and spends most of the time in a bed is certain to develop pneumonia at some point. I talked Meryl into getting up a couple of times today. Each time she was able to clear her lungs and breathe easier. But her lungs, especially the right one in which the tumor exists, accumulate more fluid each day. Can't seem to get her to try to do what needs to be done to help bring up the phlegm. Just after Dan had stopped in about midday, Meryl had a real sanitary disaster. I cleaned up and laundered all the bed linen. So I'm doing now what Meryl did for our children as infants.

Dan and Susan came over tonight, as well as Michele. Susan baked a vegetable lasagna for our supper which was excellent.

After everyone left, I decided I should sleep downstairs tonight because of the breathing problem. Meryl needs help each time liquid accumulates in her lung. Have thought about using a vaporizer and may do that yet. The blood pressure and temperature are okay, but pulse is over 100 and staying there.

Tomorrow, I will try to get her up as much and for as long as I can. Each day brings more apprehension and more and more of a conviction that the accepted treatments of today are not only barbaric, but an indictment of the claim of progress against cancer.

I am beginning to realize just how many X-rays, MRI's, Cat Scans, and so many other tests have been done. When I look at the pain and apprehension from all this, along with wondering if these tests don't cause more suffering, I have to believe that so much is not necessary. No matter what the tests show except for the blood tests, there seems to be no treatment that will help.

I'm hoping tomorrow will be a better day. Antibiotics end tomorrow, no radiation treatment or shot, so anticipate better times. The future is today and no longer tomorrow.

* * *

DAILY RECORD X

August 25, 1996

I'm convinced Meryl's hip is getting better, but lung problem is going the other way. Her condition improved in the hospital because, I think, she couldn't smoke. Now that she is home, she is smoking again. The lung is getting congested repeatedly, and she is coughing up more and more phlegm.

If there is any good news about that, it's that the color is gradually turning white again instead of the darker color it has been since the Metaport came out.

Wrote a letter today to the doctor at the San Diego clinic. Sent it along with about twenty pages of records. I also spent some free time taking window air conditioner out of her room and washed the windows.

Lunch was warmed up leftovers, but her appetite at this point is not very good. Did some more paper work in the afternoon while sister-in-law was here visiting. Shortly after, Michele arrived and stayed while I went to her house and put together the outdoor grill we had given her for her birthday. Could now put another one together in probably half the time, but this one took me over four hours. Took the proper tools, making it easier, but instructions were not too great. Michele stayed for supper, then left to prepare for her business trip tomorrow to Florida. She will return Thursday.

Just finished putting wife to bed. Gave her medication. I tried to take her temperature, but thermometer only showed 96 degrees after about four minutes. Realized that she had just taken water with pills and mouth was cold. Felt her brow and decided temperature was normal. She now is bedded down. I have chair and other equipment next to bed so she can't get out during night.

Am having a problem of my own. All at once, cigarette smoke is starting to get to me. Have put a deionizer in the bathroom which is helping. I am wondering about her temperature. Thought that oxygen was cooling her mouth and tried taking temperature with thermometer under her arm. Got a better reading. Hospital nurse previously could not get a good reading. My thought is that her temperature is below normal and seems to be staying there. From what little I know and have read, this could mean that her immune system has dropped.

She seems to be getting a little worse each day, which is a departure from previous times of chemo. By now, she ought to be feeling much better.

August 26, 1996

I found Meryl sitting up in a chair and very much disoriented this morning. She thought it was still last night. She took no breakfast except for about three sips of tea. Michele stopped by on her way to the airport, headed for Miami.

The ambulance arrived about 10 a.m. for the routine trip to the medical facility for radiation. We got Meryl on a stretcher and into the vehicle. She was on oxygen. We had a delay today. They also discovered her oxygen saturation was only about 84%, so they ordered oxygen for home use.

After we returned to the house, it was after 2 p.m., I put her on oxygen equipment the fire department had loaned me. I quickly went to the post office, and got back just minutes before an oxygen company arrived with equipment I had ordered. They left two emergency bottles, but oxygen for normal use is produced by a machine..

Meryl was not hungry, but took a couple of sips of diet coke, with cream cheese and crackers. I put up a sign reading, "DANGER, OXYGEN, NO SMOKING", where she could see it.

When Michele talked to the doctor today, he said they had done all they could and he felt it was time for Hospice care.

At this point, I'm convinced that over $75,000 of conventional treatment has done nothing to cure the ailment. The only course left is to try the San Diego clinic if she is able to travel. Right now, that's not possible. I mailed the clinic a packet of information. After the doctor reviews it, he will telephone me with an opinion.

I have been reflecting on all the information I have put in these daily messages. In a way, I am thankful I did. I've gone back several times to get dates and other data that I wouldn't have been available to me if this record did not exist. It's really not a comfort, though. I become more fearful each day.

I conferred with two radiologists at the hospital today about Meryl's condition. Prognosis was not good, but they said they would continue to try.

Ambulance arrived on time at the house this morning to take her to the hospital. I found I could move her on a chair from the bedroom door to put her on the stretcher. They were late again at the hospital, so the ambulance had to leave and return when the radiation was finished.

Returned about 1:30 p.m. and got wife back in bed. She ate a little chicken rice soup, caffeine-free Coke and Jello.

A short time later, she called me. When I reached her bedroom, she was out of bed, but it was too late to reach the bathroom. I had given her a laxative prescribed earlier and it had acted quicker than expected. It was quite a clean-up job, including bedding and carpet. Sister-in-law arrived as I was in the middle of all this, and helped me finish. She and Meryl recalled how they had done this for kids for so long. Wife smiled and said, "where are they now".

Sister-in-law prepared dinner and stayed while I was able to do some yard mowing at the apartments. Finished about 8:15 p.m. I hadn't expected to get it finished.

Earlier in afternoon, because Meryl had eaten so little during day, I fixed her a chocolate milkshake. She was enjoying it when Michele called from Miami. Also earlier in the day, I made Meryl a footstool and covered it with light blue plush carpet left over from one of our apartments. I thought she could use it to prevent the long step she had to take to get in and out of bed.

She got up before supper and spent some time in living room before going back to bed about 9 p.m. She had a bowl of ice cream and ate it all.

Even though she still is on the drug, Oramorph, which is a morphine-based pain killer, I had to give her some breakthrough Roxanol. The latter acts very quickly and, by the time it wears off, the Oramorph begins to take affect. Have set up a vaporizer in her room which I run during the night. It shuts off automatically when water gets low.

I worked on extending the oxygen tubing because the machine that makes oxygen is very noisy. I put it out in the hall, away from the bedroom, and ran tubing overhead.

So now, another day is done but have I improved anything?

August 28, 1996

Days are becoming very repetitious and ever more distressing. It's about 9:10 p.m. and just put spouse to bed. Will check again in about an hour to see if she needs breakthrough pain killer.

Nurse arrived this morning and had much trouble getting blood. When she left, there was a black-and-blue knot on Meryl's left wrist the size of a walnut. Nurse said it would go away by tonight.

The ambulance crew today included two women, who struggled, but wouldn't let me help. One was about six foot tall, sort of chubby. They were nice, and concerned. Got back just before noon, which was really early. Doctor gave me a prescription for an expectorant, but it makes Meryl drowsy and a little high.

Her chest is really becoming congested. I think it is because she is out of bed very little and is mostly on her back, as I've said many times now. Each time she sits up, she seems to get better. I am trying to force liquids down her but not getting a good response. Today she drank probably the equivalent of perhaps two and a half glasses of water. She needs to drink at least twice that much to flush out kidneys, liver and congestion.

Received a call from Dan and Hospice people are coming out Friday to discuss the situation. I'm not sure that is a good time. Not only do we have radiation then, but we have an appointment with the doctor at 1 p.m. It will be very difficult to get back by 2:30.

Dan and Michele can get all the information and let me know later. One of my brothers called tonight and said he had heard a news announcement today about the University of Texas Medical School coming up with a promising cure for lung cancer. He said they had tried it on several terminally ill patients, and apparently it has worked. If this is true, they will be swamped with calls. But I've read so many of these over the years, and it seems that little comes of the claims for cures.

I think wife's appetite is a little better, but still far from the required nourishment. Will go back downstairs in about an hour and see if she needs pain relief.

And so, another day. She still has swelling on the arm from blood taking this morning.

August 29, 1996

Noticed today how the leaves are really starting to come down. Even the maples are beginning to turn but I think it because of lack of water.

Today started like so many others, except the ambulance was about fifteen minutes late. I worried about getting to hospital late, and having to be delayed there an hour or more. As luck would have it, we got there only about five minutes late, just as the earlier patient was finishing. Meryl was able to go right in, and we were home before noon.

Lethargy has increased, except that tonight, she seemed to revive for a short time. Believe pain in fractured right hip has lessened, although I don't think she realizes it.

Michele returned from Miami this afternoon and stopped for about an hour. She brought Meryl a present, a night gown from Victoria's Secret. Unfortunately it lasted only about three hours before she needed a fresh one. She doesn't seem to have any feeling or much control on bowels.

Appetite is worse today as she ate practically nothing. Have literally been forcing water down her and any liquid she feels like drinking. The amount still is far short of what is needed.

Blood results from yesterday showed a drop in red counts. Hemoglobin, hematocrit and red blood count are all just slightly below normal. However, platelets jumped up into the upper normal area. White is okay, as are most of the other results.

Until she finishes radiation treatments, red counts will be affected. So even though Epogen shots normally are given on Monday, Wednesday and Friday, gave her one tonight and will give another Monday. That will get back on schedule. Meantime, continuing the ferrous sulfate, 384mg daily.

Tomorrow morning will be the usual radiation treatment at 11:15 a.m., then have to wait until 1 p.m. for appointment with oncologist. Bandage is to comes off where Metaport was removed and stitches will have to be taken out.

Later in the afternoon, we have the meeting with Hospice people. Dan and Michele will be there. If we are late getting back from hospital, I told them to go ahead and fill me in later in day. Hardly any appetite for supper and Roxanol again before going to sleep.

This time, the combination of radiation and chemotherapy, plus heavy medication, are leaving just a shell of what she was. I am still hoping her will is strong enough to overcome all this destruction to her well being, even though it is supposed to help. She is getting so tired. Worse, I'm afraid she also is getting tired of the battle.

August 30, 1996

Oncologist told me today that in addition to small cell lung cancer, Meryl now has "non small cell lung" cancer. I was not told how they got that information. Have seen no reports indicating this. I wonder if it came from the last transfusion. If cancer is an infectious disease as some doctors have claimed, then that could very well have been the source. Food right now is a matter of really only feeding myself, as she is hardly eating anything at all. That happened the last time she had radiation, so it looks like two weeks or so before some appetite is restored. Right now, she is surviving on the weight she gained when she had her appetite back.

Ambulance picked us up for radiation treatment today. For the appointment with the oncologist, they put her on a moveable stretcher, where she mostly slept until doctor came in at 1 p.m. At one point she awakened and said she wanted to go home, but I refreshed her memory of why we were there. We reminded the doctor about the stitches to come out, but no one had told him. Again, lack of communications.

The doctor put a softener substance on the stitches after removing the bandage. A nurse later took out the stitches.

During the session, the doctor prescribed a device which delivers a medicine by inhaling. I had planned to go to Wright-Pat to pick up the prescription plus several others. Can not get away until Sunday because there is no one to stay here. We left the hospital and arrived home about 3:15 p.m. Long day.

Dan and Michele were both here for the briefing by a representative from Hospice. We will have to look over their material and decide. About 6 p.m., a delivery man brought an inhalation device and explained how it worked. After he left, I went to do some errands while Michele stayed.

Dan had left earlier to take Susan and the boys to see an outdoor play in Chillicothe, Ohio. He left so quickly he forgot to take his suit jacket, which contained his wallet. I hope he doesn't need credit cards, money, driver's license, or anything else in the wallet.

Dan was on the television program, Current Affairs, tonight. His father-in-law called to suggest I tune in. I was too late. I'm sorry we missed it, but the nurse from Hospice was impressed and asked for his autograph.

Michele gave Meryl her supper of which she ate hardly anything. However, she is taking her medication. We literally force her to keep taking sips of water.

August 31, 1996

Meryl is hardly eating, but I think pain in fractured hip is improving. Dan called this morning and wanted to know if I was going to Wright-Pat today. I told him I thought I would have to wait until tomorrow because of Michele's busy schedule today. Dan volunteered to stay, but wondered if I would be back by 3 p.m. I explained it would depend on when I left. I told him, however, about the urgency of getting the new prescription that would allow her to inhale a medicated mist into her lungs.

We both agreed I should leave today. There was a delay of one hour on the prescriptions at Wright-Pat, so I went to the commissary and picked up a few items. Back to the clinic and prescriptions were ready, except for two. They were out and, one of them was the main reason for going. Headed back and arrived home about 2:45 p.m. Dan was surprised that I was back so early, but I didn't waste any time, other than the wait for the prescription.

I went to a local pharmacy to pick up the special medication, returned home, set up the equipment for the first treatment. I learned in a call to the doctor that the schedule for inhalation treatment is in the morning, at bedtime and one or two times during day. They should be no closer together than six hours, he said.

The doctor stopped several items of medication that were causing problems to develop. I think the stoppage was too soon from the standpoint it is better to get off drugs gradually rather than all at once. So while talking with the doctor, he agreed, and we continued the medication on a reduced basis.

I received some additional oxygen tubing I had ordered through the mail from our oxygen supplier. I used it to rig up another line to the living room. If Meryl decides to get out of bed and go into the living room, there is an oxygen connection there now. Have sort of engineered a number of things to accommodate her needs. So now, all is quiet, wife is ready to go to sleep and I have reached the end of another day.

September 1, 1996

I received an early alarm ring from Meryl this morning and hurried downstairs, but found nothing wrong. She wanted to know where everyone was. I explained it was Sunday morning and everyone probably was home in bed.

New responsibilities include the oxygen machine and the mini-compressor which powers the inhaler. The latter takes a lot of time, fifteen minutes or so each treatment, then another twenty minutes both to set up and clean afterwards.

Meryl is eating less all the time and not getting out of bed except to potty, which isn't very often these days. She is gradually getting dehydrated and fluid in her lungs is increasing.

She is becoming belligerent and demanding, and now is blaming me for not leaving her alone. She apparently believes I keep threatening her. However, we are all amused when she asks me why I am hovering over her. I understand all this, but it is still hard to accept. She really does not realize what she is doing. Her hip is improving each day and she hardly notices pain now, but that may be because of heavy medication.

Mentally, she expects pain whenever she moves. Yet several times, she has gotten up by herself and I have found her either on the bed potty or in the bathroom. The rigged oxygen lines give her as much mobility as she wants. Michele is with her now as I write this. Thought I would get started writing now and finish later.

Wife is almost asleep now. All medication is completed, equipment washed and clean. She ate a little with Michele's urging. A bite of mashed potatoes, beets, liver and onions. But that's more than she's been eating. Hope it's a sign of improvement.

September 2, 1996

Patient was not good all day. Her breathing is becoming very labored in spite of the fact that she constantly is on oxygen. She will not

302

eat and does not want to take medication. We believe that radiation is really affecting her whole system.

Michele is coming over to help with laundry tomorrow. I am hoping that with three days off from radiation, this is the Labor Day weekend and the department is closed, Meryl might recover a little from the effects.

Dan's son Riley called me tonight and wanted to know if I would come out and pick blackberries with him. Told him I would try. Dan came over about 1:15 p.m. and told me to go take care of some errands. When I got back, Michele was here and told me Riley had called twice while I was gone. She stayed while I went to Dan's house.

Dan has a four-wheel drive Honda, so Riley got on the back and Susan put Nicholas in front of me. Unfortunately, we found most of berries had dried up. What few we did find, Riley ate most of them except for two or three that Nicholas was able to swipe.

I stayed for a bite to eat and then decided I should not delay longer than the two hours I had been there. Riley didn't want me to go and started crying. I promised to come back next weekend, but he was still crying when I left. Nicholas is saying a few words, such as Paw Paw, Ma Ma and Da Da. I asked Riley if he was going to start school this year and he told me he was not going. No urging on the part of Susan would get him to change his mind, but that will change.

September 3, 1996

Not a good day, but then days seem to be deteriorating more and more. Schedule went well this morning, ambulance was early and got to hospital early. They took her into radiation about five minutes after we got there, so we were back home before noon.

Ambulance guys carried her to bed. She has been there all day, slept most of the time. Michele got here about 4 p.m. and I was able to leave to go to store for about a half hour. When I got back, Meryl was asking for more oxygen. I turned up machine to three liters instead of the normal two.

When I took her vital signs, her blood pressure was up and pulse was way up. It was about 144 beats per minute. She was also hot, skin was dry. I suspected the real problem was dehydration. I had to tell her the truth, as well as the consequences, if she didn't cooperate on what we had to do. The main thing was to immediately start a large intake of liquids, mostly water.

In about an hour, she had taken about one and one-fourth glasses of water. As it was being absorbed, the pulse gradually began coming down. In about ninety minutes, it had dropped from 144 to about 120. I am hoping this continues. Otherwise, it will mean an emergency squad trip to the hospital, where they will immediately start her on an IV. She needs to drink at least another three glasses of water between now and midnight. It means I stay up with her to see that we get as close to that as possible.

Meryl is not eating or drinking, and now is even rebelling against taking medication. Today, she's eaten a couple pieces of cantaloupe, a little ice cream and not much else.

I have been reading about some of the drugs prescribed for her and I am a little alarmed at the long-term side effects. What point is it to feel better, if in the process your vital organs are destroyed? Also, have found that some anti-depressants can become addictive and can cause mental problems. Doctor has her on a huge daily dose. Have gotten very little done today.

Received a phone call from an old friend who was scheduled for prostate cancer surgery three years ago. He told me about contacting a doctor in Washington Court House who practices alternative medicine. The doctor put him on Laetrile and a special diet. He no longer has a prostate problem and cancer is gone, he said. When he asked me to call the doctor about Meryl, I assured him I would do so tomorrow.

September 4, 1996

This has been a most hectic day, as well as night. Dan went home last night while Michele stayed. I went to bed about 10:30 p.m. while Michele stayed downstairs with the idea of sleeping on the couch in the living room.

Great breathing problem a good part of night. Before going to bed, I gave her an inhalator treatment, but kept it down to just over five minutes.

My buzzer went off about 1:30 a.m. I immediately rushed downstairs. Michele was up with Meryl, who could hardly breathe. I got dressed and called the emergency squad after talking with doctor. The doctor felt she should not go to the hospital as they would probably put her on a respirator. Her Living Will said "No" to this. We took her anyway. The emergency squad got here at 2:15 a.m., and arrived at the hospital at 2:50.

Michele had called Dan, who had been in bed only about an hour. He and Michele drove down to hospital while I rode in the ambulance. They took X-rays of lungs, put a tube down into her lung, but made no effort to get fluid out of lungs.

They gave her some medication through an IV, and told us there was nothing more they could do.

The ambulance picked her up about 7 a.m. and we headed for home. Or at least we started. But then, we were told that they could not leave until they had something in writing saying if her breathing stopped on the way home, they would not be required to resuscitate her in violation of the Living Will. Even though I told them I had power of attorney and this would not be a problem, they maintained they needed it in writing from the doctor. We waited about a half hour until they got what they needed.

She was gasping for air when we arrived home just before 8 a.m. We made her as comfortable in bed as possible, and took turns sitting up with her.

Meantime, we found that our wills, which we had made up a number of years ago and were with a local law firm, could not be found. Dan contacted a friend who made up a quick will for both myself and wife. Two of our neighbors were witnesses.

I later fell asleep sitting beside my wife's bed.

She could not be awakened during the day for medication. Except for two pills earlier, no drink and no food all day, or even now at 9 p.m. Dan insisted that I go to bed and rest, which I did in mid afternoon. For some reason, even though it was about seventy-five degrees in the house, I could not get warm. I was under the covers, even over my head and still chilled. I awakened about 5 p.m. and feel better now.

Even though Meryl still is in sort of a semi-coma or just asleep, she is breathing much easier. Instead of taking oxygen through her nose, she is breathing with an open mouth. The only liquid she has taken was mostly through an IV early this morning at the hospital. The oncologist has told us to avoid moisture and liquids, while the radiologist says the opposite. So I decided to follow my own advice and hooked up vaporizer early this afternoon. I think this has really helped, as she is breathing almost normally now.

So looks like long night ahead. Hospice representatives are coming out first thing tomorrow morning. Nurse also is coming to take blood.

September 5, 1996

Situation has deteriorated very rapidly. Meryl now is in a semi-coma, no food for two days, very little water and fluids building up in her lungs. My guess is that kidneys and liver are failing. I stayed up with her a good part of the night, although I fell asleep briefly. Hospice came in today and most of day has been a parade of nurses, social workers and others. Driveway has been full of cars the entire day.

Dan went home last night, but Susan and Michele both stayed. They have others taking care of the boys. Now it is only a matter of time. Projection is that it could be just a few hours or at most, a couple of days.

It is very difficult for me to watch her suffer. She seems very fearful and not able to move. Pulse is up as high as 150 and has not been below 120 for two or three days. Don't know how long one can survive under such circumstances. Am certain now that my intuition about the last round of chemo was correct. I am convinced now, but the decision was hers. Also, I'm convinced that perhaps blood transfusions had something to do with such a rapid decline.

She was really feeling the best she had in months prior to the last round and then, two days after transfusion, the decline began.

Michele and Dan have both taken time off from work, as has Susan. If I ever am in a situation such as this, and I have told Michele and Dan, nobody will ever put me through what she had gone through. I will add this to my Living Will.

The doctor who wrote a book on his alternative treatment called me today and asked if I could bring her to his office. When I explained her condition, he said it was too late. Somewhere in the conversation, I got the feeling he was asking me why I had waited so long. At this point, looking back on what has occurred, *I wish I had it to do over again.*

If others are going through the same thing, they need to know what the medical profession, knows but is not telling patients or family. If I hadn't read the letter that the oncologist wrote, I would not have known he projected life of four to eleven months, and less than five percent of people in this situation survive up to two years.

All these records document exactly what happened from day to day. I only wish that I could have had this experience to read in the beginning. To go through all this and to leave the world under such terrible conditions is in my mind, a form of barbarism not consistent with the progress of our society. Nor does it speak well of the medical profession, which seems to treat such things in such an abstract manner.

Guess my state of mind tonight is not too great. In a way, the sooner her suffering is ended, perhaps the sooner my constant grief will end. So much of it is connected to the terrible pain of watching her gasping for breath and not being able to do anything on her own.

How can anyone feel we have become enlightened when this phase of medicine brings only pain and suffering with little or no hope of any quality of life?

I have told those who say they share my grief to grieve for her, not for me.

September 6, 1996

Slept beside Meryl's bed all night. Condition had worsened and breathing was very difficult. Susan fixed some breakfast. We all went out to kitchen to eat. She went back to the bedroom while we were eating. I heard her call for Dan, then Dan called Michele. I knew something was wrong. By the time I got back to bedroom, she was lying there with her eyes wide open staring at ceiling. Moving a hand over her eyes had no affect.

Having watched my father go through his final hours, I felt that end must be near. I had a dream during the night in which she had made a miraculous recovery, but the light of dawn did not confirm my hopes.

I was overcome with grief at one point and had to go out in the hall. I was gone perhaps thirty seconds, then went back into the room. She had stopped breathing, and had passed on to be with the angels. Her pulse continued beating for a short time. The exact time of leaving this world was 10:35 a.m.

Later in morning, a nurse came out from Hospice. She did what she had to do to confirm death, disposed of narcotics and took some information. A social worker came out to try to lessen the grief.

But Meryl passed away peacefully, although breathing with great difficulty, with her family around her. People from the funeral home came later to take her. I made my last visit with her. We made an appointment for 3 p.m. to discuss arrangements. We decided on cremation, with a memorial service to be conducted by Father Robert Scheur.

We had company all day, and the house was full. Food has come in so fast I don't know where to put it. Refrigerator is packed full. Mitch, my brother, and his wife stayed with me until after 10 p.m. One of my former sergeants who regarded Meryl as a second "Mom " came about 9 p.m. and stayed for about an hour.

Michele came back about 10 p.m. and will spend the night here. Said she didn't want me to be alone. When I assured her I was all right, Michele said she wasn't sure she wanted to be alone. She is sleeping downstairs on the couch.

Time is now 11:40 p.m. I am tired. Guess my tears have dried up for now, although I keep saying *if I had just known in the beginning what I know now,* I would have done many things differently. After months of being on duty twenty-four hours a day, all at once all the responsibility has been lifted. Yet, so much to do before funeral service next Wednesday. We've decided to establish the Meryl R. Abraham Memorial Scholarship Fund at Ohio University, asking for contributions to the fund in lieu of flowers.

She has left this earth, and also her suffering and despair. She was fearful of death to the very end. Now, she knows the peace of moving to a better world, that is now lost in the joy of being with the angels, another world in which there is no pain, no suffering and only the happiness of being reunited with so many loved ones. And so my dear, as your spirit flies to the heavenly world that has been promised, leaving your pain-racked body in the world in which you spent 71 years, we know it is only a matter of time before you will be joined by the loved ones you left behind. May Almighty God Bless you and keep you.

The end came this morning at 10:35 after weeks and months of suffering and pain. Finally, my tears are drying and the hurt diminishing. I am not my normal self for the time being. But the void which has been left is at times, more than I can bear. Michele and Dan have seen me cry for the first time in their lives. Yes, my tears are dry for now but I know that there are many more to come. It is difficult for me to talk about this to anyone without choking up. At times, I am unable to talk at all. It is strange though, that much of my sadness comes from remembering her suffering, much more so than the normal feeling of loss when a loved one passes on to a better world.

The more I think about what comes after our life on earth, the more I am convinced it is such a change from what we now know - no more sadness, pain, greed, selfishness, competition, fighting - none of the conditions to which we succumb here on Earth.

She has gone on but I know that she cares about us and watches for our safety. In her passing, she has helped me feel such a great confidence in both the mystery of life and death. As they lifted the sheet in which she was wrapped, I realized that the shell which she has left behind no longer has meaning. It is but the earthly remains of the person with whom I had spent the greater portion of my life. The spirit of Meryl, my wife, has gone on to eternity where one day, we will all be. The loneliness I feel is but a material manifestation of life on earth. The joy she feels with perhaps a little sadness at the grief she has left behind will add to that which permeates the heavens of which she is now a part. My wife of 44 years, God bless you and keep you until we meet once more.

September 7, 1996

Slept well until about 6 a.m., then could not go back to sleep, except for a few lapses of about 5 minutes each. Got up finally, brushed teeth and had some juice and fruit. Then emptied dishwasher with Michele helping. After that, phone was kept busy with my calls going out and, in between, calls coming in from relatives and friends. As one friend told me. he didn't think that the chapel would be large enough to seat all the people. It holds about one hundred and fifty people, and I am beginning to think that he may be right.

The more I think about the medical procedures that have been utilized, the lack of communications between doctors and staff, the more I'm convinced that there is a lack of ability to organize and provide continuity. Doctors don't seem to talk with each other except, for procedures specifically requested, in which case, reports are supposed to come back to the person making the request.

Other doctors involved are not consulted nor do they make an effort to become informed. So what it appears to be is a bunch of people who call themselves professionals, all conducting their own procedures, which are based on their own opinions. Nor do I believe that reports get much attention except those which someone specifically requests for a special purpose. I'm convinced that I am more aware of what has transpired than any other person. Certainly, the hospital records have become quite thick and contain a great deal of information. But if anyone has scanned them thoroughly, it would be a surprise to me. Now, it is about 11 a.m. Need to wash up and shave. Then it is time to get a bite to eat even though I don't feel hungry and feel like anything eaten will end up in my throat. But once the food is swallowed, it seems to behave, although my stomach constantly feels tight.

Michele and I had lunch together and I ate as though I was starved. So must have been hungry. Shortly after 1 p.m., Dan, Susan and Riley arrived. Nicholas was with Susan's mother for the day. Michele and Susan left to pick out flowers for service. It will be in a chapel here in Gahanna at 1 p.m. Wednesday.

Meryl spent a lifetime with kids and it seems appropriate that the effort be continued with a scholarship fund. Through this, her concern about people will survive. About 3 p.m., Riley wanted to be taken for a ride on my tractor, so we took off. I let him steer and we rode for perhaps 45 minutes. Brother Mitch and his wife arrived, and were amazed to find him driving. Riley saw them and gave a thumbs up signal. I thought they would burst.

Later at supper, Riley announced that I should find a new girl. We all nearly dropped our teeth. When Susan asked him where, he said, "I don't know, maybe Sam's Club". Talk about emotional release.

That four-year-old kid must have super intelligence. He is certainly much more perceptive than I ever imagined. Guess he understands what has occurred better than any of us thought. Through all this, my greatest fear has been what to tell him when he sees me and asks, "Where's MiMi". But I guess I've forgotten that at his age, the impact is not like it is on those who are older and understand the finality of death.

There is a lost feeling of something very vital missing and, of course, it is the loss of my wife. After nearly 44 years of living and sharing good and bad, difficult times and pleasant ones, stress and relaxation, having someone always there or the comfort of knowing that someone was there, all at once, that comfort is gone but the love stays. And so, the feeling of missing that beloved person is not easily diminished. Only time, and a great deal of it, along with a very active life, will heal the hurt. Even the thought of her pain and suffering being

310

over, finally being taken to that world with the angels, knowing that her departure will one day be joined with mine, the happiness of the beginning of a new life, all of these reasons for joy, still do not heal the hurt of knowing that her time on earth and with her family have been called to an end.

And so, life must go on, but I find it difficult for now, to provide that comfort and assurance to family, friends and relatives, while my own emotions go out of control without warning. This, in turn, affects the emotions of others who depend upon my strength to reinforce theirs. Throughout my lifetime, I've always been able to keep my emotions under control. This time is the first major exception of my life.

The strength I've always been able to pass on to others is missing. And it will take time to numb the pain of her passing. There is so much to remind me of her, her love of life, family and especially her grandsons. And never was she happier than when she was on the beach next to the ocean, walking or lying in the sun.

In my remaining days, it will be important for me to remember the terrible lesson I have been taught by what I consider the greatest tragedy and sadness of my life. It is already so terribly lonely without her, but my grief lies in more than just her passing. My sorrow is that as she became aware finally, and too late, of what was reality and what was artificially implanted in her mind, that there was nothing I could do to reverse what had happened.

My greatest sorrow is that she should have had at least ten more good years to experience the zest of life she so much enjoyed. And I blame myself for not trying harder and understanding better what I now know I should have done and understood.

The answer was to help her look once more at life as being fulfilling as a result of her own existence. That is all gone now. It is time for me to reinforce my own faith in myself and God. For at a time when joy and sadness seem to conflict, I must believe that she is now in a far better world than any of us have known. Her suffering and pain have ended and that as she enters Paradise, she is looking down on all of us, with resentment toward none and love for all.

So I must say good-bye for now to my wife of nearly 44 years, the mother of my children and the one who sacrificed whenever it was necessary for her family and children. We will miss you and hope that one day, we will be in Paradise with you. Good-bye my beloved.

September 8, 1996

It's a little after 10 p.m., and finally I'm alone. Someone has been here since shortly after I got back from Mass. No time to get anything done that I had thought about doing. Terrible to be unappreciative about well meaning people, but there is so much to do before Wednesday. After that, legal matters, notifying Social Security, Army finance and several other agencies.

The house is packed with what came out of her office. I have been able to put some things away, but much is still out, covering a great deal of floor space. Am not going to be concerned about it until more important details are resolved.

Tomorrow, we are going to put together a board arrangement of pictures and flowers. Urn will be there with ashes. Brother Ray from Athens called and is sending a special floral arrangement that he designed. He taught art until he retired a couple of years ago. Since he is family, told him to go ahead. We just don't want a lot of flowers lining the floor. Also, would like what would be spent on flowers to go to the scholarship fund.

Papers published obituary which I had typed up Friday. Will also appear tomorrow in two papers, The Dispatch and the Athens Messenger. Had never realized that The Dispatch charges for obituaries. The one for Meryl is to cost about $400 for running two days. Preparing a tape of the music for Wednesday. Will alternate between her favorite hymns and music of the past, which she loved, such as "Moon River", "I'll Be Seeing You", "Moonlight Serenade" and "String of Pearls". Will alternate these with "How Great Thou Art", "Ave Maria", "Rugged Cross", "The Lord's Prayer" and others.

We are making up an hour-and-a-half tape which should be enough to get through the hour before the service and another half hour for the service itself. If we need more, can start tape over.

There are those who might shudder at the thought of what we are doing but memories are both joyful and sad. And departures are also a time of joy and sadness, joy because the trial of living our mortal lives has ended and now going to a better world - sadness because of the void that is left for those of us who have to stay behind for the time being. Had about an hour and a half this morning after Mass to myself so sat down and began writing book that I hope will help those who have to go through our experience. It is something that I wish I could have had at the beginning and certainly, *what I have learned would greatly affect what I would have done had I known then what I know now.*

So even though I had to spend much time in reading and research, that information and experience would have been so valuable to me if I had known in January. It will always be one of my great regrets in life. If there is one thing in life that does not change, it is the guilt that hindsight brings. It is with great emotion that I hope that what I write will reduce the feeling that I have felt and am feeling, that of *"If I had only known in the beginning".*

September 9, 1996

It is 11:15 p.m., and the last neighbor just left. Am really tired tonight. Turned on computer about 9:30, doorbell rang, and it was neighbors who somehow discovered that I was alone tonight. Problem was that I was looking forward to getting to bed. For some reason, and it was also late when I got to bed last night, woke up about 3:35 this morning and couldn't go back to sleep.

So got up and watched tutorial on Windows 95. After eating a bite of roll and some juice, started getting tape ready for Wednesday. By 10:30 a.m., had about thirty minutes finished out of a ninety-minute tape. Several selections are by the Norman Tabernacle Choir. Some had to be taped from CD player, which I don't have, so Dan borrowed one this afternoon. I finally got it finished about 5:30 p.m.

A lot of time was used up with Michele and Susan wanting some of their music but they first had to listen to all of the music. Just to give you an idea, it took the better part of the day to make the original tape. They all wanted copies and it took me, after they left, about an hour and a half to make three copies of the original. Problem is that as I listened to some of the music, emotion got the better part of me.

After family left, thought I would have some time to do other things. However, between phone calls and visits, had very little time to myself. Some friends with whom I've not had contact for several years and no address or phone numbers turned out to be easily found.

Have a program on my computer which can find anyone in the US if they have a phone. Was able to find everyone and reached all of them except one. There was no answer and no answering machine so will try again tomorrow. Now, it's 11:30 p.m. and I am tired. Sort of keyed up also, but after I brush my teeth, will probably go to sleep pretty quickly. Was able to maintain better control of myself this evening but it will take awhile. Forty-four years is a long time for such a sudden change.

September 10, 1996

Got up this morning after waking up the first time about 3 a.m. From then I dozed on and off. Woke up finally and got up about 6:30, took a bath, soaked in warm water for about ten minutes, finished, shaved, etc., and got dressed. Had a few things to do. But what I did was without thinking and awareness.

Later in the morning, Dan came over and printed a map of how to get to his house. He invited everyone to come there for food and drink. I think that enough food is coming in to feed an army. Can't believe how many people and how much of it.

We left about noon to take some stuff out to Dan's house, then to rental place to pick up a special table to use at chapel tomorrow. The table that was ordered somehow was no longer available so rather than put ourselves in jeopardy by making a decision for Michele and Susan, we put things on hold until they could be reached and make the decision.

Dan dropped me off at home about 2:45 p.m. Got in the car and went to three grocery stores before I found a couple of hams. Told them I would bake one for tomorrow and ended up buying two. They were small and with both being just over seven pounds, a total of fifteen pounds. Turned off the oven about 7:30 p.m. and, as they cooled, tasted one. The taste met the test. Guess I still have not forgotten as these are first hams I have baked in several weeks.

House smells hungry too. While hams were baking, neighbors brought in a huge tray of meat, etc., cake and huge cheese ball. Had to really repack the refrigerator in order to empty one complete shelf to put in tray. Can't believe that I got everything back in. They stayed for about a half hour and then left. Two women and a man. He is a retired colonel and an old friend of mine.

Got quite a few sympathy cards in the mail today so I guess people have seen the obituary. Several people have called to say how nicely written it is. How does one write something like that nicely

Michele just called to tell me that her roomy in college just arrived with spouse. They are staying with her tonight. So, as soon as I send this message, will bundle up hams and take them out to Dan and

Susan's. Her mother is going to get there early tomorrow morning and will slice up the hams. Time is now about 9:30 p.m. so should get back by 10:30 p.m.. Then to bed and will hope for a solid night's sleep for a change.

September 11, 1996

There are so many regrets about so many things but what is hurting me most are thoughts of the last days and how scared she was of what was happening to her. Also, I had hoped for one more Christmas, but that will not be. So Christmas will never be the same again, as she made it an event, because of the joy she has always felt for her children and grandsons.

But perhaps this all happened so that I could put it all together in print so that others who will or are going through the same experience will have a better understanding of what will happen or is happening. They won't find out from the medical profession and, in truth, they take the attitude that putting people through such terrible treatment is doing those who suffer a favor. But enough of that for now.

Got up this morning after getting little sleep last night, had some juice, a roll, a banana and vitamins. Finally got through to Social Security Administration and found out that the earliest that I can make an appointment to make necessary corrections is in October. Got dressed, etc., hadn't heard from anyone and by 11:55 a.m., was about to leave for the funeral home. I was getting a little concerned about whether details had been completed.

At that moment, Michele arrived with her former college sorority room mate and her husband. Then Susan got here and they both went into the bedroom to change. They had been at the funeral home and didn't want me to have to be concerned about details.

By the time we got to the chapel, friends had already arrived. Went inside and they had done a beautiful job of putting things together, pictures, flowers, etc. Was surprised at the number of flowers as we had asked that they not be sent. They put the tape on the music system and got immediate compliments from several people. I never got further than the entrance to the chapel until just before the service started.

People were coming in. The line got so long that it stretched outside the door and stayed that way for over an hour. Couldn't believe how many people came. In the hour, perhaps nearly 300 people stayed in line for quite some time. Ran out of parking space and people began parking on the grass. Then that ran out and some people were unable to come in.

Father Schuer arrived, but I didn't know that he was on heavy medication in preparation for a sonic breakup of a kidney stone this coming Friday. Still, his service was touching, but he kept pronouncing Meriam instead of Meryl. Everyone knew how particular she was about how her name was pronounced, and finally, someone mentioned it to him. Michele had a poem she read, and she pointed out nothing had changed with the name pronunciation.

Father Scheur later asked me why he erred and I reminded him that he used to do the same thing. She would constantly correct him. After the service ended, and conference with funeral home personnel, we went to Dan's house. There must have been 50 cars. But I guess many had already left. My fifteen pounds of ham went almost immediately. So many people from so many places, some of whom I hadn't seen or from whom I had not heard in a number of years.

Meryl must be pleased as she looked down on the events of the day. Now, there is nothing more I can do for her, except pray for her soul as God gives her a place in heaven among the angels.

* * *